BEAUTY
AND
MEDICINE

BEAUTY
AND
MEDICINE

Robert Aron-Brunetière

Translated from the French
by Joanna Kilmartin

JONATHAN CAPE
THIRTY BEDFORD SQUARE LONDON

First published in Great Britain 1978
Jonathan Cape Ltd, 30 Bedford Square, London WC1
Translated from the French *La Beauté et la médecine*
© 1974 by Éditions Stock
English translation copyright © 1978 by Jonathan Cape Ltd

British Library Cataloguing in Publication Data

Aron-Brunetière, R.
Beauty and medicine.
I. Beauty, Personal
I. Title   II. Kilmartin, Joanna
613'.0424   RA778
ISBN 0-224-01449-8

Printed in Great Britain by The Anchor Press Ltd
and bound by Wm Brendon & Son Ltd
both of Tiptree, Essex

Contents

Illustrations

Diagrams

Tables

Foreword

No dermatologist should ignore a book on the skin which is already a 'best seller' in another country. One simply had to be interested because it was likely to increase public demand for one's professional advice. However, when I first read Dr Aron-Brunetière's *La beauté et la médecine* my immediate reaction of delight was followed by acute anxiety.

In 1969, having spent almost fifteen years as an apprentice in British dermatology, I did a world tour, visiting as many clinics as possible. I learned that everywhere dermatologists were better trained to provide beauty treatment than I was. I watched acne surgery in Boston and Sydney, teenagers 'prepared' for a ball in Munich, and went with colleagues to Warsaw and Prague on their evenings in cosmetic clinics. Later I visited an acne clinic in Miami where teenagers went through a routine of documentation, education and treatment which was quite unlike anything available in Britain. I have many friends in the U.S.A. and France who give as much time to beautifying the skin of their patients as does Aron-Brunetière, but while I am not short of friends among British dermatologists, I know of none who practise in this way.

It is, of course, entirely normal to wish to be attractive, and if one picks up the majority of women's journals, there is no shortage of information although not all of it is accurate. One must welcome this book because on the common issues it is full of information, acceptable to dermatologists, and more understandable than most of the information provided for patients by doctors.

The public is very ready to receive such information and herein is the worry! Only a few years ago the government of this country was still hoping that every need of every person would be met by an increasingly sensitive service. Some ministers even expected it all to be free. Unfortunately there are many people who have been brought up to believe this and cannot equate it with economic truths. As a dermatologist who is a member of a Community Health Council – the watchdog of the National Health Service that voices public opinion about health matters – I see how difficult it is for the layman to make a list of priorities. I fear that many readers of this book will expect to receive more care of the skin than is in fact available. Aron-Brunetière suggests that small dilated blood-vessels in the legs should be treated by electrolysis as early as possible, but even if they have severe varicose veins most people have to wait for one or two years for professional help. In France there is one dermatologist per 50,000 of the population but in Britain there are only about 200 dermatologists and the government will not allow more than a ratio of 1 per 197,000. About 50 dermatologists do private practice part-time and there are a few full-time private practitioners who will provide help for the paying so-called 'privileged' minority. It is possible to have face-lifts and hair transplants if you pay for them, but the facial peeling described in this book as a regular service is very scarce indeed.

The development of the Psoriasis Association and Eczema Society has at last provided a voice of the consumer which governments are prepared to listen to. Some established dermatologists have been very suspicious of these patient organisations but most have begun to realise that in a country where the professional has no time to meet even serious demands, laymen can themselves organise a great deal. The Red Cross Beauty Care and Camouflage schemes are a splendid example. Many organisations will certainly welcome this book because on the one hand it provides advice and describes how one can help oneself and, on the other hand, it vividly outlines the fears and distress of those afflicted with abnormal skin. Hopefully the realisation that there is a demand for care of a kind that probably never will be free, will help to silence the awful cry for the total abolition of private practice and a totally free National Health Service. Those who wish to spend money on making themselves attractive by buying the services of experts may be allowed to do so, as in Warsaw and Prague. Aron-Brunetière gives a balanced view. He warns those who want to spend their money not to give it to charlatans. He speaks to the establishment, telling them to regard the cosmetic as a scientific discipline. This reminds me that when I wanted to send a member of my junior staff on a tour of European cosmetic clinics, the 'Dermatological Establishment' was opposed to it. It would not look good at the appointments committee!

Of course, no dermatologist would agree with everything another recommends and there are fashions in prescribing which some are quicker to follow than others. In contrast to many dermatologists, Aron-Brunetière hates comedone extraction but uses hormone creams, injects embryo and placental extracts and believes that rosacea is due to allergy. Allergy is not fashionable but immunology is and no doubt in a few years we will know whether or not they mean the same thing.

Aron-Brunetière communicates and communication is in vogue. Because he is a Frenchman and I am an Englishman, we differ on the emphasis on the harmful effects of sun or cold. English women are appallingly stupid about clothing in winter. While this book is good on dieting and exercise, the harmful effect of smoking is omitted. Smoking is never beautiful.

Perhaps I have said enough to explain why I think there are many who will welcome this book but still more who will notice how little we are equipped to meet its demands.

T. J. RYAN,
Consultant Dermatologist

The Slade Hospital,
Oxford

Introduction

It has become an obsession. One must be young, one must stay young. Youth is the dominant cult of our time. It means not only protest, demonstrations, covering the walls with graffiti, tearing up paving-stones, fighting the police, growing your hair long if you're male and cutting it short if you're female, but also a market to be exploited, a market in which industry invests millions in clothes, cosmetic 'lines', records, for whom advertisers rack their brains in order to think up new styles, new fashions: skirts up to the thighs one minute and trailing on the ground the next.

And everyone else follows suit, desperately trying to keep up. If to be young is to go to extremes and act the fool, then plenty of adults qualify. But to be young is more than that: it's not only being able to rebel, to say 'Make love, not war', to laugh at taboos, to refuse to be trapped by systems, to challenge age-old assumptions: it's having firm muscles, supple joints, healthy arteries and a sound heart. It's not necessarily to be beautiful, for youth is by no means always beautiful. One can be beautiful at any age.

Youth is in no sense a prescription for beauty: it cannot be attained by aping the young. Especially as each day that passes brings us closer to the time when we shall be wrinkled, rheumaticky, short of breath ...

Is there nothing to be done then? Must we resign ourselves to the effects of wear and tear, decrepitude, disintegration? Quite the contrary! We can prevent paunches, combat bulging thighs, delay and minimise the ageing of the skin, raise sagging breasts. The means exist, we have only to make use of them – though I hasten to add that it is probably more often a question of avoiding mistakes than embarking upon treatment.

What treatment?

I hear people complain that they have tried all manner of expensive cosmetics with little or no result.

That is not what I call treatment. For a doctor, treatment signifies the various means, whether hygienic, medical or surgical, which can be employed to preserve or restore health and which possess clearly defined, scientifically tested properties enabling them to be correctly applied in order to achieve the desired result.

In most spheres of medicine, this definition applies to all forms of treatment.

In dermatology, however, there were until recently two separate classes: diseases of the skin, where the above principles strictly applied, and those disorders which, because they only affect the looks and do not constitute true diseases, were regarded by traditional dermatologists as unimportant. Indeed, anyone who suggested that they merited attention was liable to be considered a charlatan by other members of his profession.

But what justification is there for dermatologists, whose function is not only the diagnosis and treatment of skin disease, but also its prevention, to dismiss its common disfigurements as unimportant? The fact that they are not true diseases? But we know that a simple rash may be the prelude to eczema, just as a common cold may be the prelude to pneumonia.

What is the justification for their indifference to the consequences of the vast sale of creams, lotions and other cosmetics to tens of millions of consumers? The fact that cosmetics are associated with vanity and frivolity? But cosmetics are not inert substances; they can and do provoke skin reactions. A spiritual asceticism in accordance with which we should hold our miserable fleshy envelope in contempt? But it would be equally true to say that the care we lavish on it is a way of honouring the Lord by respecting and cherishing his work. A hangover from the days when medicine was too preoccupied in saving what could be saved with its limited means to have the leisure to bother about anything else? But those times are past.

I remember a lecture given in 1935 by my professor, René Leriche, one of the greatest surgeons of his day, in which he told us that the average life-span in a country like ours was fifty-four years. Today, it is seventy-three or four — a gain of twenty years in less than forty!

That has made all the difference; inevitably, our attitude to human existence has changed, and with it our attitude to human illness; and this change was bound to break down the barrier between the two classes of dermatology.

Various trends in this direction have emerged over the past

twenty years, but the turning-point was not officially reached until 1972, when the agenda of the International Congress of Dermatology included a general discussion on 'dermato-cosmetology'.

For dermatologists of my generation, the introduction of cosmetic dermatology in the agenda of an international congress was a revolution. It meant that dermatology was coming down to earth, was at last coming to grips with everyday reality, and would no longer be able to pretend to ignore it.

But this revolution was really the result of a gradual change in the attitude of patients themselves, who brought to our consulting rooms, as well as their ailments, an awareness of their right to health, to physical and moral well-being (the two are inseparable) and an increasing and justified conviction that their internal condition was not everything and that external appearance was important too.

In other words, it was the patients who were the revolutionaries: in terms of medical treatment, we now have a 'consumer revolution', as the economists would say. And this revolution has obliged doctors to rethink their methods of practice and their relationship with patients, as well as imposing new responsibilities on them such as informing the public: it is no accident that doctors are increasingly in demand on radio and television, that more and more articles are published in the non-technical press about new developments in medical knowledge, which has advanced more in the past thirty years, thanks to the progress in the related sciences of physics, chemistry and mathematics, than at any time since man first appeared on the earth.

If ordinary people are to make the most of this progress, they must possess a minimum of knowledge in order to be able to judge for themselves and make choices. This is not to say that it is essential to understand the laws of energy in order to make use of electricity, or that a woman must know what an ultra-violet ray is before she goes sun-bathing. Nevertheless, there are certain things we need to know about electricity – that it can kill, for example, if you use the telephone or shave in the bath – and about the sun – that it can seriously contribute to the ageing of the skin.

But here we come up against a problem which is, I believe, central to our day and age: that of communication. I mention it now because it is a problem I shall face throughout this book, since what I write is designed to inform a reader who is not necessarily

B

equipped to receive the message I hope to communicate, always supposing, in the first place, that I am capable of making myself understood. Watching certain television programmes, I have often thought that my colleagues, despite their admirable and manifest efforts at simplification, were having difficulty in 'getting across'. Nothing is more difficult than to simplify matters which are the reverse of simple, without falling into the trap of over-simplifying to the point of distorting the facts.

I have experienced this myself when being interviewed live on television; I did my utmost to make myself understood, and I have no idea whether or not I succeeded. There is no escaping the fact that each scientific discipline has its own vocabulary, so esoteric as to be inaccessible to the layman. I understand nothing, or next to nothing, of the vocabulary of mathematicians, nor they, as a rule, of mine.

Doctors are sometimes accused of using 'big words' which ordinary people cannot grasp. This is said to be either a way of concealing their ignorance (which was true in Molière's day) or else a means of domination: and it's certainly true that a fluent and assured manipulation of words which are above the head of the other person will succeed in giving him a sense of inferiority and making him uneasy, even anxious. But 'connective tissue' is connective tissue; there are no other words I can use to describe it. On the other hand, I can explain why it is called that, where it is and what its functions are, and I shall not hesitate to do so, because it is one of the essential elements of the skin, playing a part in the formation of wrinkles – and wrinkles are important.

Scientific terminology is not made abstruse or complicated for the sadistic pleasure of men deliberately setting themselves apart from their fellow-men out of vanity. It is applied to objects which have no equivalent in everyday life, and designates them either by means of familiar words used in a different sense from the normal, or else by specific words which have no other usage. Together, these words make up an esoteric vocabulary which medical students must learn and, once they have qualified, use to communicate with one another.

But it is not simply that medical terminology is out of the ordinary; there is also the question of how it is used, of a special way of thinking. A medical report has nothing in common with fiction: it is a cold, concise, impersonal statement of facts which are then analysed and discussed; there is no place for circumlocution or purple passages. Doctors, like researchers — and many doctors are researchers — are taught that facts are paramount, regardless of personal opinions, which must always be subordinate to them. The scientist must always be open-minded, and prepared to question his own conclusions. From this point of view, he seems to me to be the antithesis of the politician; I could not imagine a party politician who constantly called his party's doctrine into question or hesitated to make the facts fit his opinions: he wouldn't last long if he did!

I mention all this to show how difficult it is for people with this sort of training — one might almost say conditioning — to break out of it and communicate with the outside world about matters connected with their specialist field.

There are those, it is true, who look down on the world from their pinnacle of learning and refuse to descend to its level; their specialist knowledge is their own affair, their monopoly; the masses can simply take what they are given without asking why, and be grateful.

Others, without being in the least arrogant or condescending or contemptuous, are often no less reticent, because they are afraid of being misunderstood or misinterpreted. And that is why they are wary of journalists.

I don't, of course, mean those journalists who specialise in medicine and who are, for the most part, doctors themselves: they do an excellent job of popularisation; and even those who are not doctors do their best to assimilate complicated questions and then communicate them to the public without distortion or inaccuracy; and on the whole they do it intelligently.

Unfortunately, this is not always the case: in 1952, I published, together with my colleague Dr E. Sidi, a book entitled *A Summary of Corrective Dermatology*. The aim of this work was to indicate to non-specialist doctors and to members of the nursing profession what they might expect from the means then available for the correction of disfiguring conditions resulting from certain skin diseases. One chapter is devoted to a particular problem in which I am a specialist, and in it I expressed my opinion on the dire effects of various external treatments which, traditional though they were, should in my view be abandoned. A women's weekly magazine mentioned the book and this chapter in particular, and for some mysterious reason the journalist responsible wrote the precise opposite of what I myself had written. This caused me endless trouble: for the next two years I had a succession of patients who proudly announced on arrival: 'I do everything you advise, doctor.' Since they had of course gleaned their knowledge from this widely circulated magazine, the routine they were so assiduously following was in every respect the exact opposite of what I had advised.

I ended up by interviewing patients with my own book ready to hand, marked at the famous chapter, and every time a patient made the aforesaid declaration, I would read out the passage in question.

Anyone can make a mistake, and that one could have been much worse. The type of journalism doctors and scientists dread above all is that which seeks out the sensational and automatically gives it priority over more routine information, as though headline news were the only news worth printing.

Our lives are not confined to the spectacular or the exceptional; they are made up of little commonplace things that occur every day. But the fact that they are commonplace does not mean that they are insignificant, and the tiny mistake which, in isolation, would not matter in the least amounts, with repetition, to a serious error entailing the gravest consequences.

Thus I am constantly seeing people whose skin has been seriously damaged, not to say become diseased, as a result of being subjected morning and night over the years to a routine of skin-care, seemingly quite ordinary but, alas, quite wrong for them.

I am well aware that there is a large public with a hunger and a need for sensations and marvels to give them a momentary respite from their daily problems. But in the field of health, where anything and everything may be of concern to the reader, the commonest illnesses are in fact the most important: I never see any mention of cirrhosis of the liver in alcoholics, or the circulatory and cardiac disorders it causes, whereas the rare heart-transplant never fails to hit the headlines.

Five years ago, the *Cahiers du médecin spécialiste*, the quarterly organ of the French specialists' association, asked me to write an article for the benefit of my colleagues on 'the non-contraceptive effects of the pill'. The day after its appearance, a Paris newspaper carried a four-column headline on its front page saying 'The pill does not cause cancer, says Dr Aron-Brunetière'. It is true that I had written, *inter alia*, that current investigations tended to exonerate the pill from the suspicions surrounding it (subsequent research has confirmed this: the incidence of cancer of the uterus is lower among women who take the pill than among those who don't); but my article also revealed other facts which were of practical interest to the general public: for example, that certain brands of the pill constitute an excellent treatment for female acne. Only that wasn't considered sensational enough, and no one thought it worthwhile singling out and writing about.

I need hardly emphasise that the sensational has no place in the information which this book will attempt to provide. It is not an encyclopedia of beauty, nor does it contain any recipes for beauty-aids. It will certainly disappoint anyone with a taste for the arcane and the supernatural, or who believes in the magical virtues of products deemed to be 'natural', as though the fact of being natural were a guarantee of beneficence and harmlessness.

We forget that dear Mother Nature scatters our woods and fields with over twenty varieties of wild mushrooms — natural enough, in all conscience — the least deadly of which have toxic effects that cause vomiting and violent diarrhoea, whilst the worst can destroy the kidneys or the liver, produce hallucinations or delirium, coma or death.

Opium, that deadly drug from which morphine and heroin are derived, is a completely natural product which leaves an unending trail of violence, bloodshed, and physical and moral collapse; hemlock, the poison with which Socrates killed himself, is no less natural; and the same is true of curare, with which the South American Indians smear their arrows in order to paralyse their enemies, and peyotl, the Mexican cactus which secretes mescalin, an alkaloid with hallucinatory properties similar to those of the notorious LSD. The list is endless, from the tropical timbers which cause eczema among workers in timber-yards to the only too natural nettle. Examples of this kind would fill a book.

The approach to beauty has as little to do with such elementary ideas as it has with the idea of poets or women's magazines. It consists mainly in the acquisition of technical knowledge without which one cannot understand why such and such a thing must be done, and such another avoided, why one thing is feasible, another not; the knowledge, in short, which is needed in order to preserve or create a personal style of beauty.

I say personal because beauty is a many-sided concept; the dictionary defines it as: 'that which arouses feelings of admiration or delight', a definition which does not, in fact, mean very much. Indeed, this feeling of admiration and delight depends to a very large extent on the prevailing notion of beauty; and this notion has always varied from age to age, from place to place, from one civilisation to another, according to personal taste and the symbol it evokes: the generous curves of Juno, mother of the gods of ancient Rome, represent a very different form of beauty from those of the boyish figure of Diana the huntress.

Beauty presupposes harmony of proportion and volume; yet its 'canons' — that is to say, the unit of measure which serves as a 'module' for sculptors in determining the proportions of their statues — have often varied from one artist to another. For the sculptors of ancient Greece the beauty of the foot depended on the second toe being longer than the first, whereas for the ancient Egyptians the length of the toes had to descend in decreasing order from the big toe. We admire the body of the Venus de Milo, but it seems unlikely, to judge by Rubens's heavy-breasted, broad-beamed women, that she would have delighted the burghers of seventeenth-century Flanders. Certain black African tribes equate beauty with the length of the neck, elongated by means of super-imposed rings; others with pendulous earlobes, weighed down with discs; both are hideous to our eyes.

Beauty presupposes a compelling majesty which can often be intimidating in its coldness. Moreover, what is handsome in a man — an aquiline nose and chiselled features, for instance — would be thought ugly in a woman.

By the same token, to be beautiful is not necessarily to be pretty: one can be one without the other. A short person, provided she is well-proportioned and has attractive features, may be extremely pretty; but no one would say she was beautiful. Conversely, a statuesque young woman with calm, regular features, even if she is on the heavy side, can evoke, by her femininity, a kind of beauty; but no one would think: what a pretty girl.

And here we come to the crux of the problem: I don't believe that one can acquire beauty: one is born beautiful. If your parents have bequeathed you short legs, you are stuck with them for life; but you can still make yourself more or less agreeable to look at, that is to say, pretty. And it is on this level that we can act, for prettiness is determined by factors in which we can intervene directly: the contours of the body, which are connected with the muscles and subcutaneous fat; the appearance of the face, dictated by certain structures — nose, eyelids, ears, chin — which can be modified in any number of ways by plastic surgery; and the condition of the skin, which can be preserved or improved.

One does not have to be a dermatologist to know that it is impossible to be beautiful or pretty with an ugly skin, and that the skin deteriorates, fades, slackens, wrinkles — in a word, ages; that, in ageing, the prettiest skin ends by growing ugly, and that when one grows old it is in the appearance of the skin that the process first manifests itself.

I shall try, therefore, to show first and foremost the how and the why of this gradual process, in order that everyone may understand the reasons for certain rules the aim of which is to delay the process as long as possible.

For the important thing is to age well, with dignity and grace.

1 What is the skin?

Put like that, of course, the question seems childish. Naturally we all know the outer envelope which moulds itself to each of us like a body-stocking, and we would reply that the skin is what covers our body and the bodies of animals.

But this skin of ours – the source of pleasant sensations when caressed, or painful, unpleasant ones when ill-treated – is no ordinary wrapping like the peel which protects the segments of an orange.

True, like orange peel, the skin has a protective role: it isolates from the outside world that other, complex world which goes to make up each separate individual: bones, muscles, nerves, circulatory vessels, glands, viscera, in other words, what is called the 'interior environment'.

It might be described as a barrier, but a living barrier, *an organ in its own right, serving numerous functions* in addition to its protective role.

Every living thing is by definition fragile and perishable; everything which functions can break down. The skin is no exception, and because it is in direct contact with the outside world it is exposed continuously, more than any other organ, to all manner of injuries. When you consider that it is susceptible to diseases resulting from various internal disorders into the bargain, it is not surprising that its equilibrium, threatened from within and without, is precarious and easily upset. Nor should we be surprised that considerable vigilance is required to keep it in good condition; but vigilance is not enough without a minimum of foresight, and foresight in turn requires a minimum of knowledge.

The first thing I shall do is to explain what the skin consists of and how it behaves; this strikes me as all the more necessary because my patients' remarks and questions constantly reveal how misinformed, if not totally ignorant, the majority of people are on the subject.

To take one example: a woman patient was asking me about 'peeling'; peeling, as the word implies, is a dermatological treatment which involves peeling the skin. (I shall come back to it in a later chapter because for some conditions it can be a very effective procedure.)

I could tell that my woman patient (women are more interested in peeling than men, as a rule) was worried about something; it wasn't the peeling itself, since I had just explained the procedure to her in detail, and it's nothing to be alarmed about; she was worried for another reason, as I was not long in discovering:

'Do you remove an entire skin, doctor?'

'Hardly that, just a very thin layer from the surface.'

'You mean it can be done more than once?'

'But of course!'

'How many times?'

'As many times as you like, depending on the benefit you can expect from it.'

My patient seemed amazed; after a short silence she went on: 'But I don't understand, I always thought we only had seven skins ... '

I must confess that the first time I heard this remark I was flabbergasted. I've heard it often since. There seems to be a belief that the body is covered not merely by a single skin but by a reserve of spare skins as well; a total of seven, in fact. I've never been able to discover the origins of this myth about the skin whereby the magic number seven appears to have the same symbolic meaning as it has in the seven churches, the seven angels, the seven plagues, the seven-headed dragon and the seven seals of the Apocalypse.

I reassured my patient: we have only one skin which renews itself continually throughout our lives; how else could it heal and form scars?

THE STRUCTURE OF THE SKIN

This skin is made up of three distinct, superimposed layers, each closely joined to its neighbour. Beginning with the deepest layer, these are: the hypodermis, the dermis and the epidermis. Together these three layers constitute the skin or cutaneous tissue.

Here I must digress, for I've just used one of those everyday words I mentioned earlier which have been incorporated into scientific language: when I use the word 'tissue' it has a quite different meaning from that generally understood.

In the strictly biological sense, a tissue is a collection of cells possessing the same structure and functions.

And, in this context, by 'cell' I mean the basic unit of all living tissue, of every living thing whether animal or vegetable. Just as it takes countless millions of grains of sand to make a beach, so it takes countless millions of cells to make a human being.

Without cells there can be no life. The cell represents the fundamental distinction between living matter and inert substances such as minerals or gases.

Each cell is a little world in itself, a world which we have long been able to penetrate and learn about, thanks first to the ordinary microscope and, more recently, to the electron microscope with its enormous power of magnification (up to one million times) which shows every minute detail. Every living cell (with a few rare exceptions) is surrounded by a membrane isolating it from its neighbour.

All living cells, without exception, contain a central body called the nucleus; you could say that, like the stone or core at the centre of a fruit, it is the nucleus of life. A cell without a nucleus is a dead cell. If I seem to insist on this point, it is because dead cells like these, without a nucleus, exist on the surface of the skin and play a crucial part in the protection of the inner environment.

Each of these millions of minuscule worlds is bathed in a salty fluid whose salt-content is roughly that of sea-water; the interior environment is a kind of salt lake from which each cell draws the substances it needs in order to live, namely the chemicals which are its nutrients and the oxygen it must have in order to breathe. No cell can live outside this salt lake, which represents 80 per cent of the body-weight; were it to dry up, there wouldn't be much left of a man who had weighed 80 kilograms.

The cells can excrete the waste products of their respiration and digestion into this lake without creating pollution because, when everything is functioning normally, the waste products are treated in such a way as not to pollute the interior environment. Once the mechanism breaks down, however, once the cells cease to function normally in any part of the machine, then the waste products become pollutants and the organism falls ill.

The form and grouping of the cells is not the same in all tissues. These depend on the role the tissue is designed to perform and, in any given tissue, all cells work uninterruptedly at the same task so that it can fulfil its purpose properly. In the bony tissue, the cells build up the skeleton; in the glandular tissue, they manufacture the hormones. And in each of the three layers of the skin the cells also have their precisely characterised form, grouping and activity.

THE HYPODERMIS

The hypodermis is the deepest layer of the skin. Situated immediately underneath the dermis ('hypo' means under), it is chiefly composed of fat secreted by specialist cells. This so-called adipose tissue varies considerably in thickness from one individual to another and will sometimes increase to enormous proportions in obese people.

It also varies from one area of the body to another in the same individual: there are places where the hypodermis is virtually nonexistent and the skin appears to be very thin, as though stuck to the bones: on the spine and the nose, for example; where it is thick, as on the buttocks, it gives them their characteristic curves.

It also differs from one sex to the other: the distribution of adipose tissue is not the same in men as in women; it is responsible for women's rounded forms and—when not too pronounced—harmonious curves.

This fatty tissue acts as insulation, protecting the interior environment from variations in temperature on the exterior: fat people usually feel the cold less than thin people. It also facilitates the gliding action of the skin over the deeper structures when the body moves.

Lastly, the hypodermis represents an energy reserve on which the organism can draw according to need. It diminishes, to the point of vanishing completely, in cases of prolonged fasting or serious illness—hence the expression 'all skin and bone' to describe the condition where there seems to be nothing left between the two remaining layers of the skin, the dermis and epidermis, and the skeleton, every bony contour of which is visible. Unfortunately, doctors of my generation became only too familiar with this dreadful sight when examining deportees who had survived the Nazi concentration camps.

THE DERMIS

Immediately above the hypodermis is the most important area of the skin, the dermis (from which the word dermatology is derived). It is made up of a network of fibres manufactured by specialist 'fibroblast' cells. Nowhere is the term tissue more applicable than to this fibrous mass, resembling as it does the warp and weft of woven fabric, which, because of its linking role, we call 'connective' tissue.

The connective tissue of the dermis is the skin's armour-plating. Broadly speaking, it is composed of two sorts of fibres: the majority are grouped in bundles, forming undulating, interlacing bands; they are made of a special substance called 'collagen', which will produce gelatine when boiled in water. Intermingled with these is a network of other fibres which are thin, sinuous and made of an elastic substance known as 'elastin'. Although this group of fibres represents only about 2 per cent of the connective tissue, their importance is nevertheless considerable.

The blood circulates in the dermis through tiny arteries and veins and minute canals known as 'capillaries'. These capillaries are of the utmost importance because it is through their microscopically thin walls or membranes that the exchange takes place, between the blood and the cells, of the fluid or lymph on the one hand, which impregnates them as I have described above, and the nutrients and respiratory gases on the other.

The dermis also contains:

1 The sensitive nerve-endings of the skin through which we recognise the five sensations which go to make up the sense of touch: pain, light touch, deep pressure, heat and cold;

2 The sweat glands, which secrete the sweat; a fine duct takes it upwards through dermis and epidermis to the surface, where it is expelled through an opening invisible to the naked eye; this is the 'sweat pore';

3 The roots of the hair and their accompanying glands, the sebaceous glands, whose greasy secretion, sebum, or seborrhea if it exceeds normal limits, produces the oily skin and clogged hair which causes so much distress. Whereas sweat glands are found over the entire surface of the skin, sebaceous glands and hairs are not present at all in some areas, notably the palms of the hands and the soles of the feet.

THE EPIDERMIS

A thin membrane marks the upper limit of the dermis, above which is the epidermis ('epi' means above). Really a wall of cells, the epidermis contains neither arteries, veins nor capillaries; the lymph essential to the life of the epidermal cells comes from the dermis.

At the base of the wall is a continuous layer of small, cube-shaped cells quite different from those we have come across so far. Known as 'basal' cells because they lie at the base of the epidermal wall, they are the parent cells of all epidermal cells. The basal cells continuously generate new cells which pile up above them, so that the youngest cells of the epidermis are to be found in its deepest zone and the oldest on the surface. Not only are the latter old in

DIAGRAM I   Vertical section of the various layers of the skin

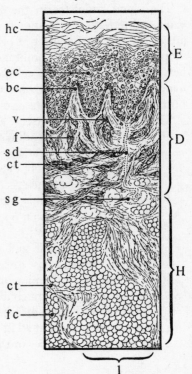

E: epidermis, with
hc: stratified horny cells, without nuclei, at the surface of the skin
ec: epidermal cells with nuclei produced by the
bc: basal cells
D: dermis, with
v: a small vessel
f: fibroblasts
ct: bundles of connective tissue and elastic fibres
sg: sweat gland and its duct (sd)
H: hypodermis, with
l: lobules of fat cells (fc) separated by septa or connective tissue (ct)

relation to the cells which have pushed them to the top, they have also aged due to the modifications they have undergone during their progress towards the open air: gradually, their nucleus disappears, they flatten and become charged with a substance called 'keratin' which eventually transforms them into a horny layer. Human nails and hair, horses' hooves, stags' antlers and the horns of cattle and sheep are all made of this substance, which can be of varying degrees of hardness.

The 'horny' cells on the surface of the skin, having lost their nucleus, are not merely old: they are dead cells. Lying in several superimposed layers, overlapping rather like roof-tiles, they cover the entire surface of the epidermis where they form its first line of defence against any substance which might try to penetrate it in order to reach the body's interior.

The most superficial of all become detached and are shed, to be

DIAGRAM II Vertical section of the epidermis, greatly enlarged

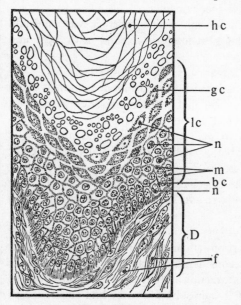

lc: 'living' epidermal cells; bottom layer: wall of basal cells (bc). Above: the 'prickle' cells generated by the basal cells with their nuclei (n), their membranes (m) and, shown in cross-hatching, the filamentous material in the cytoplasm with extensions holding the 'prickle' cells together.

As it ages, the epidermal cell becomes charged with granules (gc: granular cells); then it loses its nucleus and becomes

hc: a horny cell

D: dermis with fibroblasts (f)

replaced by similar cells from below. This continuous phenomenon is not visible to the naked eye unless it is exaggerated, as happens in a skin disorder such as dandruff: those familiar, unattractive greyish-white scales which powder the shoulders of our clothes are none other than horny cells.

Lastly, intermingled with the basal cells are the cells which manufacture pigment, or 'melanin'. These are the cells which, according to their quantity, dictate the colour of our skin — white, yellow, copper or black — and, in white-skinned races, cause the skin to tan when exposed to the sun.

THE FUNCTIONS OF THE SKIN

The cutaneous envelope is responsible for a number of functions, one of the most important being the regulation of the body-temperature by means of:

1 The protection afforded by the insulating properties of the padding of fat in the hypodermis; and
2 Two active protective mechanisms:
   (a) the arteries of the dermis which contract with cold and diminish internal heat-loss, or expand with heat and augment it;
   (b) the secretion of sweat.

As we know, what distinguishes cold-blooded animals from warm-blooded animals is the fact that the body-temperature of reptiles and fish is linked to the temperature of the outer environment, whereas the body-temperature of birds and mammals is independent and invariable regardless of external heat or cold; within certain limits, that is: too-intense cold or too-great heat can overtax the regulating mechanism and cause death. In very hot weather, the sweat helps to cool the surface of the skin through its evaporation.

Together with the kidneys, the skin also plays a part in the elimination of the waste products of cellular activity, in particular of urea which exists in considerable quantities in sweat. There have been serious cases of uraemia and fever in art schools because students who had painted themselves all over had succeeded in completely blocking their sweat-pores.

Lastly, the skin represents a barrier between the organism and the surrounding environment which can be breached from within by substances such as urea, as we have seen, or salt (sweat is salty), but never, under normal conditions when the skin is healthy and intact, from without. In other words, if I may be allowed a deliberately exaggerated simile, the skin operates in the opposite way to the fence surrounding a prison camp through which you can enter but from which you cannot escape.

This is not to say, however, that the skin is totally impervious: true, water cannot penetrate it (which is just as well for us, otherwise we would swell like a sponge every time we had a bath), but in special circumstances, such as prolonged contact or when irritated, certain products can cross the epidermal barrier provided that they are small enough or soluble in the fats on the surface of the skin.

We exploit this potential in medicine, where some medicaments can be administered just as effectively by rubbing them into the skin as by injection; but it can also have undesirable effects, as in the case of substances which produce an allergic reaction.

This brings me to the end of an indispensable piece of homework; without this much background knowledge, it would be impossible to understand how the skin lives and evolves, why it reacts badly in some conditions and well in others, or why certain procedures or applications are ineffective, others harmful, and yet others essential.

THE CLASSIFICATION OF SKIN-TYPES

According to the classification largely popularised by women's magazines, there are only four types of skin: normal, dry, oily, or 'combination'! At first sight, this may seem clear, precise and straightforward; but until we know exactly what is meant by these adjectives, they tell us nothing. And it's in trying to explain them that difficulties arise.

Clearly, if a skin-type were so obvious and simple to define, women wouldn't be in such a state of uncertainty; they would have no need to go to a beautician or a dermatologist for advice.

When they do so, incidentally, their approach can vary considerably. I find that patients normally ask: 'What's my skin like, doctor?' meaning: is it good or bad? In this case the patient is asking for a diagnosis as well as reassurance; she doesn't have preconceived ideas, she wants a specialist's opinion so that she knows

c

where she stands and what can be done. She's prepared to listen to what he has to say and abide by his verdict.

But there's another, very different approach. 'What kind of skin have I got?' isn't at all the same question. It implies: which category do you put it into? This patient likes to put things into pigeonholes; curiosity having got the better of anxiety, all she really wants to know is her position in the scale of values laid down by her favourite weekly.

And in some cases I am even presented with a ready-made diagnosis: 'I've got a combination skin, doctor.' This is a categorical statement, the patient hasn't the smallest doubt that she has a 'combination' skin, sometimes she even knows that her skin is 'dry and oily at the same time'; how this can be, I've no idea, but she knows it for a fact, just as I know that I'm going to have my work cut out with her, for no one is harder to deal with than the person who thinks she has all the answers; she's suspicious, obtuse, deaf to reason and impossible to help. She hasn't come to consult me in the ordinary sense of the word, to ask me for a diagnosis and, if possible, treatment. Quite the contrary! She already has her diagnosis: she wants to know what I advise for her 'combination' skin; but no doubt she has her own ideas on that subject as well, and it never occurs to her that she may not know what she's talking about.

Such attitudes can be carried to extremes. I was treated to a glaring example a few years ago by the bossy, domineering mother of a spotty teenager. Sickly, pale, narrow-chested, shoulder-blades sticking out, the poor girl was hunched up and visibly overwhelmed by this hard-faced woman who had dragged her all the way from the depths of the country to see me. Throughout our interview, or I should say her mother's monologue, I never once heard the daughter's voice; before I could say a word, the mother had launched into a long speech designed to explain for my benefit the symptoms exhibited by her offspring and her opinion as to their cause, winding up with a detailed description of the treatment I should undertake. There was nothing left for me to do except to write out the prescription.

But not even thirty years of practising medicine have inured me to such pretentious displays of half-learning and, inevitably, I lost patience. The good woman must have been baffled and indignant when I told her that, honoured as I was that she should have taken the trouble to come so far to give me the benefit of her wisdom, she had, alas, chosen the wrong man; not only was I too pig-headed to profit by it, I so profoundly disagreed with her interesting views that we might as well consider the consultation null and void.

Thinking back over the years, I don't see what more I could have done. I still feel sorry for the daughter, who was badly in need of help; but I could have given it to her only over her mother's dead body!

It shouldn't be assumed from all this that a doctor wants his patients to come cap in hand, humbly to gather the fruits of his knowledge. On the contrary, I'm convinced that no doctor can do his job properly unless he establishes a dialogue with the patient, and no patient will follow a treatment conscientiously unless he or she understands why it has been prescribed and what can be expected from it. This means that the doctor must make the effort to explain and the patient to understand – but for that, he or she must be receptive, amenable and without preconceived ideas.

And how disastrous these preconceived ideas can be: vague, ill-digested notions spread by word of mouth or picked up from newspaper articles which give the illusion of being authoritative. Today, medicine belongs to everybody and everybody has his own set ideas about medicine. People put us to the test: 'Doctor, do you know about this new cancer treatment?' or else they advance their own theories: 'I know someone who found that such-and-such a treatment worked, don't you think I ought to try it?' The answer is that, yes, we do know about the 'new cancer treatment', which isn't new at all, as it happens; and no, unfortunately the treatment which worked so well in your friend's case won't do for you because it's for hives, and not everything that itches is hives: you've got a type of eczema, which is quite different ...

Of course, we don't know everything. Nobody does. But each of us tries to keep abreast of events in his own field. And that means continually adding to one's knowledge by hours of reading every week in addition to normal work. Anyone who doesn't choose to make the effort will find himself out of date in six months, so rapid is the advance of knowledge today. The result is that this techni-cian we call a doctor, who is learning his job every day of his life, who has the modesty to recognise his limitations but who also knows what he is capable of, doesn't suffer dogmatic **opinions** gladly, especially when expressed by people who disseminate false ideas with an air of authority matched only by their ignorance. Doctors get impatient when they hear about a 'combination' skin, for example, the amazing conjuring trick whereby you can have two different, contradictory types of skin on the same face, 'dry and oily at the same time'. Such trendy jargon is rubbish, it doesn't mean a thing. It has generally been dreamt up by some publicity man who wants to create a grandiose-sounding formula to impress the public and persuade people to buy the products it is his job to sell. It bears no relationship whatever to reality.

The usual classification of types of skin into normal, dry or oily is far too generalised to give more than a sketchy idea of the subject. Of course it can serve as a point of departure and, indeed, that was my original intention: to take these three categories and describe them, one by one, in the usual way.

On thinking it over, I came to the conclusion that I would not only bore the reader but myself into the bargain, and that, personally, if I happened to have an oily skin—something I could see for myself without being told—what I would want to know would be why.

Clearly, in order to tell at what point a skin ceases to be normal, and to understand why this happens, we must first be able to recognise the characteristics of normal skin and the combination of circumstances which must exist if it is to remain so.

NORMAL SKIN

It may be surprising, but there is no such thing as a definition of normal skin. Like a contented people, its history is uneventful, and therefore tends to be ignored. Nevertheless, we are wrong to ignore it because experience shows that this normality consists in a precarious equilibrium which is constantly being threatened by many different factors.

The popular assumption that a normal skin is one which is neither oily nor dry is meaningless, technically speaking. It's a truism, like saying that a normal skin is one which is not abnormal! The completely normal skin exists only in a healthy child before puberty. Typically, it is firm, because the supporting connective tissue is dense and solid; it is supple, because its elastic fibres are numerous and in excellent condition: when you pinch it, it doesn't wrinkle and quickly regains its shape; it is fine-textured, smooth, without visible pores and velvety to the touch; it is matt, because it secretes very little sebum; and, lastly, it is clear, seeming almost transparent in fair-haired people, because of the harmonious relationship between the various factors which to go make up the complexion or skin-colouring.

There are three such factors:

1 The pigment, which governs the amount of brown, from pale to very dark, in the skin: the reason dark-haired people's skin is never completely white, as it is in fair or redheaded people, is because it contains a greater amount of pigment and consequently tans more easily when exposed to the sun;

2 The thickness of the horny layer, which accounts for the grey in the skin: the thicker it is, the greyer and muddier the complexion;

3 The circulation of the blood in the tiny capillary vessels in the dermis, which gives the skin its pinkness. A contraction of the blood-vessels causes paleness, whereas if the vessels dilate, the increased flow of blood causes the skin to flush. This is a well-known reaction in shy or emotional people who easily become 'covered in blushes' and sometimes intensely red over the entire face and chest.

The skin of a healthy child, which is a miracle of perfection and glowing freshness, is fated to undergo certain changes at the onset of puberty, that important phenomenon, that turning-point of life when childhood is finally over and, by way of adolescence, adulthood looms ahead.

HORMONES AND THE SKIN

These changes are linked above all to the appearance around this time of significant alterations in the glandular secretions. From birth, even while still in the womb, we possess a group of glands called the 'endocrine' glands which secrete into the blood substances which they have manufactured. These products are the 'hormones'.

Everyone at some time has come across a reference to hormones; indeed, since the advent of the pill, they've been constantly in the news. However, if the truth were known, I doubt whether many people understand the precise nature of these highly specialised substances which govern our general well-being from the beginning to the end of our lives, are sometimes at the root of serious, even fatal illnesses, and play no small part in determining whether we are beautiful or ugly to look at.

The glands which produce the hormones constitute the endocrine 'system', just as the brain, the spinal cord and the nerves constitute the nervous 'system'.

There is a close link between the endocrine and nervous systems: this isn't surprising when you consider that the brain governs our entire body, so much so that a person cannot be considered dead until it can be proved that the brain's activity has ceased.

The relationship between nervous and endocrine systems is controlled by a gland called the *pituitary* which is attached to the base of the brain by a little stalk.

The pituitary gland has a number of functions: it controls growth by virtue of a special type of hormone, a deficiency of which causes dwarfism; it produces another type of hormone which acts upon the pigment and yet another which dissolves fats; finally, it has under its sway, like a conductor his orchestra, all the other endocrine glands:

1 The thyroid gland, whose swelling causes goitre;

2 The suprarenal or adrenal glands, which sit above the kidneys like a three-cornered hat and secrete, among other substances, the cortisone which is essential to life and those hormones related to the male hormone;

3 The pancreas, which secretes insulin, a deficiency in which leads to diabetes;

4 The parathyroids (four glands lying to the side of and behind the thyroid gland), which regulate the amount of calcium necessary to build up bone;

5 The sex glands, testicles in men and ovaries in women.

I have mentioned only a few of the more distinctive characteristics of these glands. In fact, there are many more types of hormones than this deliberately short list might indicate, and each one usually has several functions; this results in an extremely complicated mechanism whereby certain functions are carried out by several types of hormones acting in concert, whereas others are controlled by different types acting in opposition.

Until puberty, the sex glands are at rest. From puberty onwards, their activity is controlled by the pituitary gland:

The testicles begin to secrete large quantities of male hormones which will cause the voice to break, the pubic hair to grow and the sexual organs to enlarge.

The ovaries begin to manufacture two types of hormones: one is the female hormone proper, oestradiol, of which oestrogen is the most active component; the other, progesterone, prepares the uterus to receive, as into a nest, the egg or ovum once it has been fertilised by a spermatozoon. Together the female hormones control the development of the breasts and the onset and subsequent rhythm of menstruation which will normally occur every twenty-eight days until the menopause.

In addition to these visible effects, the sex hormones have several other, less immediately apparent effects, especially on the skin: male hormones cause the epidermis to thicken and the sebaceous glands to enlarge, stimulating them to produce the fatty substance we call sebum or seborrhea. They also possess the tiresome property of causing the scalp hair to fall out.

Unlike male hormones, female hormones reduce the thickness of the epidermis — which is why women's skin is always thinner and less robust than men's — restrain the activity of the sebaceous glands, and have no effect on the hair. On the other hand, they control the distribution of fatty tissue in the hypodermis that gives women, more generously endowed in this respect than men, their typical roundness of cheeks, thighs, hips, buttocks and shoulders; in short, the curvaceousness associated in our minds with the beauty and softness of the female form. It is by cramming themselves with female hormones that male transvestites, who reject their male state, manage to alter their subcutaneous fat and acquire female contours.

Female hormones also have the property of dilating the blood vessels and, for this reason, women are especially prone to a number of congestive conditions: varicose veins and broken veins of the cheeks are much more common in women than in men, who also never suffer from those networks of red or purple capillaries which have such a depressing tendency to spread over female calves and thighs.

Lastly, female hormones are responsible for the water retention which occurs in all women just before their periods: normally slight, a few hundred grams at most, it is neither troublesome nor noticeable. But it can become an obsession in women who find that, for several days every month, they feel heavy, swollen and uncomfortable.

The effects of male and female hormones on the epidermis, the hypodermis, the hair, the sebaceous glands and the blood-vessels can therefore either be appropriate (in which case they are called specific effects), or quite inappropriate.

In the dermis, on the other hand, their activity is directed towards a common end: male and female hormones alike stimulate the manufacture of the connective and elastic fibres and in this way help to maintain the tone and suppleness of the skin in both sexes.

Once puberty is over, the skin's equilibrium, its normality in other words, thus depends to a considerable extent in both men and women on the normality of the hormonal secretions of the sex glands.

2 *Oily skin or seborrhea and its consequences*

I've just been explaining all this to Annie D. Annie is eighteen years old and has come to see me because she has an oily skin. With her greasy hair hanging in strands, and glistening face, she looks rather like a wet dog. Like most of my young patients (those, that is, not accompanied by a chaperon who answers all my questions in their stead), she has listened seriously and attentively to what I have been saying. She quickly proves that, as I thought, she has taken it all in.

'You mean that the reason I've got an oily skin is because I possess male hormones?'

'Exactly.'

'But women don't have male hormones!'

'That's a perfectly intelligent response. All the same, Annie, they do. Just as a normal man produces minute quantities of female hormones, so a normal woman produces minute quantities of male hormones. Men never suffer in consequence, nor do the majority of women, because the amounts are too small to affect the hormonal balance.'

THE MALE HORMONE AND THE FEMALE SKIN

'However, in some cases – and they are by no means rare – overproduction of the male hormone, a condition we call "virilism", will cause certain organs in women, the skin in particular, to develop masculine characteristics; this "masculinisation" involves the appearance of seborrhea, the thinning of the scalp hair and the development of body hair. When I see a woman with seborrhea or thinning hair, the first thing I do is to establish whether she has any abnormal body hair.'

'I've only got an oily skin, nothing else.'

'That's true, your condition has nothing in common with the extreme case I've just described, the kind of condition which is accompanied by serious hormonal disorders. Seborrhea can exist on its own, without there being any over-production of male hormones.'

'Now I'm confused; you seem to be saying the opposite of what you've just told me.'

'That's because I haven't had a chance yet to explain everything to you in detail. Try thinking of the endocrine system as a manufacturing industry in which you have producers and consumers. In this case, the glands which manufacture male hormones are the producers and the sebaceous glands which use them are the consumers. Let's say that our product is wine: among consumers of wine are people for whom a single glass, a normal, reasonable amount, is enough to make them drunk — they are abnormally sensitive to alcohol. In the same way, there are people whose sebaceous glands are abnormally sensitive to the effects of male hormones and who get "drunk" on quantities which would leave other people quite sober. These people can develop an oily skin without there being any over-production of male hormones. In other words, women can have seborrhea whether or not they produce an excessive amount of male hormones.'

THE MALE HORMONE AND THE MALE SKIN

'What about boys?'

'The situation is different with boys because by definition the production of male hormones is at a maximum; in other words, there can't be over-production. Indeed, when we measure the quantities of male hormones present in boys some of whom have seborrhea and not others, the amounts secreted are always found to be the same; consequently, masculine seborrhea can only be the result of a malfunction at "consumer level".'

THE ORIGINS OF SEBORRHEA

Sometimes puberty can come and go without mishap; the skin preserves the well-balanced look and clear complexion of childhood because everything is functioning perfectly — hormonal production is being kept within bounds and the sebaceous glands are reacting sensibly: there is a very slight, imperceptible sebaceous secretion known as *physiological seborrhea* which is actually necessary to maintain the equilibrium of normal skin, as we shall see when we come to talk about dried-up skin.

Unfortunately, for 60 per cent of girls and nearly 70 per cent of boys, things don't go so smoothly. The skin becomes shiny, the complexion takes on a muddy tinge owing to the thickening of the horny layer of the epidermis, and the pores dilate. The centre part of the face, the forehead, nose and chin, is always the first to be affected, the middle of the forehead usually being the worst. Normal, necessary physiological seborrhea has turned into *pathological seborrhea*, that is to say, an unsightly skin disorder.

With luck, things get no worse. Usually, though, the seborrhea spreads to the sides of the face. Experience shows that the earlier seborrhea appears, the greater the chances that it will become serious, persistent and difficult to treat: the most troublesome forms are those which occur in boys around the age of fourteen and in girls of about eleven. In extreme cases, the coating of sebum becomes compact and waxy: the skin resembles orange-peel, pitted with holes that can reach a millimetre in diameter with, between them, slight bulges which give the skin a quilted appearance when examined under a microscope. The whole face looks swollen, as though bloated. Left to itself, seborrhea may clear up spontaneously after a few years. It can also last a lifetime. Worst of all, it can be complicated by acne.

THE COMPLICATIONS OF SEBORRHEA

In the first instance, 'comedones' form; more commonly known as 'blackheads', they block the pores so that the sebum can no longer flow over the surface of the skin, causing it to become slightly less oily.

AN IMPORTANT SKIN DISORDER: CLOSED COMEDONES

Ugly though blackheads are, provided that one doesn't commit the cardinal error of squeezing them, they don't turn into painful, inflamed spots. Compared to what can and often does occur, they are a minor evil.

In addition to the blackheads, a different type of comedone forms in the depths of the dermis, completely enclosed by the skin. Unlike blackheads, of which they are an aggravated form, these 'closed comedones' have no opening to the exterior. While blackheads will dry up and vanish spontaneously, *closed comedones, once developed, never disappear*. They are the cause of acne pimples: indeed, closed comedones and acne spots are so closely linked that one can safely say that acne cannot exist without them.*

When a dermatologist examines a patient with acne, it isn't the spots that interest him, still less the blackheads, but the closed comedones.

The acne sufferer finds this difficult to understand: all he can see are his spots and they are all that matter to him. It is because of them that he had come for advice. If he can't produce a veritable constellation of pustules on his back and neck to show the doctor on his first visit, he gets very worried and apologises for being in one of his 'good' periods. Over and over again a patient will say to me:

'It's a pity, I've got hardly any spots today; you should have seen me a couple of weeks ago!'

He's surprised when I say:

'I don't have to see your spots in order to be able to tell how bad and extensive your acne can be.'

'Really, how is that?' he wants to know.

Spots come and go; sometimes they erupt, sometimes they're quiescent. It depends on various things: nervous tension, prolonged worry, being generally run-down. I had a patient once who was doing a body-building course. Every muscle stood out beneath his skin. He had impressive-looking biceps, pectoral muscles worthy of a Greek statue, an abdomen like steel, and everything else to match. I soon came to the conclusion that the physical effort he was imposing on himself in order to achieve these results was responsible for the waves of huge, painful, hard red lumps buried under his skin, showing beneath the surface and lasting for weeks or even months. He was suffering from what we call 'deep cysts'. But once he decided to sacrifice his 'superman' look, there was a rapid improvement.

In women, the progress of acne is chiefly influenced by menstruation: there is nearly always a fresh outbreak during the preceding week and occasionally also at the time of ovulation.

---

* Closed comedones are popularly known as 'whiteheads'. (Tr)

'I've noticed that myself,' a patient will tell me, 'but I find that it lasts longer than a week in my case.'

'That's so, sometimes the outbreak will start with ovulation and continue until the beginning of the period. And if the period is late, it will last longer still. It always calms down after the period is over, which is why the skin looks relatively clear then.

'That's why, when you want to know how bad someone's acne really is, you don't base your judgment on the spots but on the closed comedones which are their cause, their starting-point. Since closed comedones are permanent and each one is a potential spot, all you need do is to examine the skin for them, note their size and number, and you can tell precisely what sort of an outbreak of spots a patient is likely to have, and where. This can be seen at a glance, even if the patient doesn't have a single spot at the time.'

'I know I've got blackheads, because I've seen them, but I haven't noticed any closed comedones.'

'I'm not surprised; because they're so deep they're often barely visible. Look at yourself in this mirror: you need to stretch the skin between your fingers; now do you see those little white spots the size of a pinhead? In some people they're so close together they virtually blanket the skin, especially on the sides of the chin, as in your case, or on the temples, the neck or underneath the jaw. Unless they're very large they're hard to see when a patient is standing up. That's why I asked you to lie down just now, in order to examine you under a strong light.'

Seborrhea, like acne, occurs most often on the face, but it can also affect the back as far as the buttocks, the shoulders, the arms down to the elbow, the chest, the nape of the neck and the neck itself.

I've had many patients, men and women, well past the age of thirty, who have never been to a public swimming-pool or taken their clothes off on a beach because their bodies were so repellent to look at; and others who were enforced celibates owing to the smell of rancid butter given off by their skin.

This is typical of the effect seborrhea and acne can have on the social, emotional and even professional lives of sufferers; it's difficult, if not impossible, for them to get jobs which involve meeting the public, no matter how well-qualified they are: other things being equal, an employer will give preference to someone with a wholesome, pleasant appearance over a candidate with spots.

Even people with fairly mild seborrhea or acne are self-conscious about it, especially when it's persistent. And these disorders, when they persist after the age of twenty, seldom clear up spontaneously.

The oldest patient I have treated for acne was forty-seven, and he had suffered from it since he was twelve: thirty-five years of an existence dominated by spots is a long time; they can make life a misery. So much so that, except for a morose few who give up hope and rail against the injustice of fate or medicine in general for failing to help them, the majority of sufferers continue their trek from beauty clinic to homeopathic clinic to dermatologist in search of a cure which they still hope to find despite setback after setback. One can well understand why, fearing yet another disappointment, their attitude is one of scepticism mixed with hostility.

The pattern of the interview is always the same; it usually opens with the patient saying: 'You're the tenth person I've seen', and continues with: 'I've tried everything there is and you can see for yourself what good it's done me.' One can sense his tension and misery.

'Not a great deal, I agree; you've lost hope then?'

'I've got good reason to, haven't I?'

'Why are you here in that case?'

'A friend of mine knows someone who got better ... '

He stares fixedly at the ground, not looking at me. They're all the same, I can never see anything but the top of their heads.

'Would you mind raising your head so that I can examine you?'

As I scrutinise him, I can sense him watching me, waiting for my reaction.

'Lie down over there, please.'

His is a typical example of adult acne; the upper part of the face is oily but free from spots; these are concentrated in the lower part, in the area of the beard, whereas in juvenile acne the spots affect the whole face with a tendency to predominate on the forehead. The transition from the juvenile to the adult form usually takes place around the age of twenty to twenty-one.

'Do you think you can do anything?'

'Probably,' I reply (I can tell that he's thinking 'that's what they said when I was twelve years old'), 'but I'll be able to tell you better when we've had a talk.'

He relaxes slightly.

'I'm glad you didn't say yes straightaway.'

'Why?'

'Because that's what I'm told every time I begin a new treatment.'

In some cases one can be positive, in others one has to be more cautious. Certain types of seborrhea or acne can only be cured by a dermatologist in conjunction with a psychologist or psycho-analyst. And acne in men is always more recalcitrant than in women.

ACNE AND SEXUALITY

A good many of those sufferers determined at all costs to find a cure are married women and mothers who know from bitter experience that there isn't a shred of truth in the famous old wives' tale that 'It'll soon clear up once you're married'. What's so heartbreaking is that this ludicrous piece of advice is still being handed out today. The fact is that apart from a few, very rare cases, sexual activity has no effect on seborrhea. Moreover, there's no earthly reason why it should. True, the nervous system participates to a considerable extent in the sexual act, and it could be said that this affects the hormonal balance. Every gynaecologist or endocrinologist knows of cases where, due to this mechanism, a woman's periods have become normalised after marriage.

However, the influence exerted by the nervous system can be bad as well as good, as in the case of a young girl who came to me with her face, shoulders, chest and back covered in appalling acne. I learned after questioning her that this explosion of pustules only dated from a few months previously and that until then, while she had had an oily skin and a few spots from time to time, it hadn't amounted to anything much. Rather surprised by the suddenness of this change, I asked her about her periods: these seemed to be normal, and their rhythm had not altered recently; nor had she been receiving any hormonal treatment which might have upset her hormonal balance.

On the principle that there's no smoke without fire, and that seborrhea doesn't flare up to that extent for no reason, I questioned her about her parents and her job; it often happens that a patient is antagonistic towards either mother or father, or towards the people at work, or even to the work itself. This antagonism causes nervous tension and anxiety which can have repercussions on the functioning of the glands; no sooner do these rebellious individuals go away on holiday and relax than the appearance of their skin improves. Such fluctuations in seborrhea are commonly seen in students working for an exam or a scholarship, especially if they happen to be the emotional type of person who sweats more than normal: the skin actually looks far more oily when there is a lot of sweat and little sebum, than when there is a lot of sebum and little sweat.

In the case of my young patient there were no exams, she had no problems at work, which she greatly enjoyed, and she got on very well with her parents. The only remaining possibility was an unhappy love affair; but here, too, things were going well for her, almost too well. She was sleeping with her boy-friend and the only thing that marred this otherwise highly satisfactory state of affairs was that, within forty-eight hours of the first occasion, she had suffered the spectacular outbreak of spots which had led her to consult me. Had she not been living at home, this might have seemed no more than coincidence. As it was, her movements were somewhat circumscribed and she was unable to see her lover very often; by jogging her memory, it proved easy to establish a relationship between her love-making and her outbreaks of spots: each time she made love, she paid for it by bursting out in spots. It was enough to cool down the most hot-blooded temperament! I managed to cure her and, towards the end of her treatment, I confess that I encouraged her to give full rein to her feelings in order to test the soundness of the result.

This is the most outstanding example of sexuality having a deleterious effect on an oily skin that I have seen. Happily, such cases are rare, as rare as those where its effects are beneficial, and in the vast majority of cases its effects are nil—in which case the unfortunate sufferer is then encouraged by family and friends who tell her: 'You've only got to have children and it'll soon clear up.' She has one, then another, then a third, sometimes even more; and each time there is renewed hope because, after a short period of deterioration during the early months of pregnancy, the seborrhea dries up, the outbreaks of acne disappear and, until her confinement, the mother-to-be triumphantly presents to the world if not a peaches-and-cream complexion, then at least the clear, matt, spot-free skin of her dreams.

Alas, scarcely is the mother home with her baby than her complexion regains its usual blotchy, muddy, shiny look and the wretched cycle of spots begins all over again. As one unfortunate woman said to me: 'I only look presentable when I'm expecting a baby, but one can't go through life being pregnant.'

Nor need she, for there are effective means of remedying this state of affairs. Which method you choose depends on the degree of the trouble in question: there is a whole series of gradations between a skin that is slightly oily around the nose and chin and a face that glistens all over with seborrhea, just as there is between having a few little blackheads on and around the nose and an extreme case of acne.

SEBORRHEA IS A DISEASE

Moreover, the borderline between what is considered by some to be a mildly disfiguring but purely cosmetic problem and by others an actual disease is extremely ill-defined.

Where does unsightliness end and disease begin? To put it another way, at what point does a skin cease to be 'on the oily side' and become truly diseased?

Personally, I regard this kind of distinction as purely artificial: mild seborrhea means that a predisposition must exist; there is always the threat that it will get worse. To take a typical example: two women of the same age, leading exactly the same kind of lives, have fibroids. One has a normal skin, but the other has a slightly oily one and her hair tends to become greasy four or five days after shampooing; she also has down on her cheeks. A course of male hormones is prescribed for both women – the classic treatment for fibroids. The woman with normal skin suffers no ill-effects whatever. The other sees her seborrhea get steadily worse, her hair become greasy within two or three days and the down on her cheeks thicken or even give place to hairs; and she'll be lucky if, during the next few months, her scalp hair doesn't come out in handfuls.

In other words, it is easy to turn a merely unpleasant condition into a distinctly abnormal one, and it is important that mild seborrhea, even if it doesn't require the same degree of treatment as acne, should nevertheless be taken seriously and treated in the correct way.

This brings me to a conflict of opinion existing between derma-

D

tologists and beauticians. It's a rather one-sided dispute since dermatologists, who have the necessary qualifications and means to treat any condition falling within the scope of dermatology – or for that matter, if they so desire, cosmetology – clearly have no reason whatever to pick a quarrel with beauticians except when, by overstepping the narrow limits of their competence, the latter put the public at risk. (I'm referring to those beauticians who think nothing of tinkering electrically with the tiny tumours they call 'warts' – to the uninitiated, every little extrusion on the skin is a wart – whereas in reality what they are meddling with are cancerous tumours: a certain type of mole or 'beauty-spot' liable to malignant change. One can't help shuddering when one knows the mortal danger involved when the least untoward interference could precipitate the lightning dissemination of a disease capable of killing within months!)

However, this hasn't silenced the controversy over the distinction between what the beauticians call 'care' and treatment. 'We don't give treatment,' they say, 'we give beauty-care.' According to this strange logic, beauty-care, because it doesn't involve the use of medicaments, is never harmful, whereas treatment, which employs active drugs, can entail certain risks. Of course this is mere quibbling over words: any undertaking to care for or to treat an abnormal condition implies a responsibility to take the appropriate means to remedy it.

Furthermore, while it's true that the use of many drugs entails a certain risk – the price one pays for their active properties – it's quite untrue to suggest that beauty preparations are free from risk: they too possess their active properties, their so-called 'active ingredients', otherwise what would be the point of using them? And because of this they may well have undesirable effects, for the simple reason that, being chosen more or less at random, they're liable to be unsuitable for the skin destined to receive them.

This being so, the idea of separating the concept of beauty-care from that of medical treatment is purely artificial; just as it is to separate the two spheres of activity.

The fact is that the management of a skin disorder is based on the same principles whether it is mild or severe: in the first case, local, that is external, applications may be sufficient; in the second, one may need to add internal treatment; but in both cases, the local treatment is the same and the same errors must be avoided.

The best illustration of this lies in the wealth of misunderstanding that surrounds the treatment of seborrhea.

I have already described in detail the internal factors which cause over-secretion of the sebaceous glands resulting in oily skin and greasy hair.

I shall now explain how and why incorrect local treatment of the skin can either sustain or aggravate this condition.

THE WRONG WAY TO TREAT AN OILY SKIN

For more than three-quarters of a century sufferers from seborrhea have been encouraged not only to get married, but to perform a series of rites expressly designed to dry up the skin: first, a good soaping, preferably with an acid soap; next, a rub with an alcohol solution containing camphor or tincture of iodine, or else with a mixture of ether and acetone; after that, an application of an ointment or solution containing sulphur, and, for good measure, at least twenty minutes under a sun-lamp.

The unfortunate victim will persevere with this systematic assault for a month or two at most; I've never known anyone stick it out for longer. The results are always the same: the skin soon begins to burn, it becomes rough and mottled, its surface takes on a mica-like appearance, then peels; meanwhile the sebum flows inexorably from the dilated pores. What had been a straightforward oily skin is by now both oily and irritated, sometimes even more oily than it was to begin with. Once it has been burnt by the ultra-violet rays of the sun-lamp into the bargain, the picture is complete!

I've been pointing out for the past twenty years that this approach to skin care is utterly misguided, and that all products traditionally used and labelled 'for oily skin' or 'for greasy hair' should be withdrawn from the market.

During those twenty years I've had patients who would never have become my patients at all had they not actively encouraged their seborrhea by employing these kinds of remedies.

A lot can be learned from observing and listening carefully to hundreds of patients all suffering from the same complaint. It teaches one to question a number of traditional ideas.

For instance, it has taught me not to jump to conclusions and assume that an oily skin is tough just because it is thick; in fact, contrary to popular belief, an oily skin isn't in the least robust: it is fragile, sensitive, and always reacts badly to the slightest mismanagement.

I have also learned that the more you try to de-grease an oily skin, the oilier it becomes, and the more so the more determined your efforts. Every woman with seborrhea of the scalp soon learns to her cost that the more often she washes her hair, the quicker it will become oily again. If she is one of those women who are obsessed by their oily hair, shampooing it at too frequent intervals, there will come a point where it's in worse condition twenty-four hours after being washed than it was when she washed it every five or six days.

I've christened this phenomenon *reactive seborrhea.*

Any product that drastically de-greases the skin — soaps containing too much detergent or grease-solvents such as alcohol, ether and acetone — will unfailingly provoke reactive seborrhea.

Some face-creams can also have the same effect: these are the so-called 'vanishing' creams, freely available on the cosmetic counters, which appear to vanish as soon as they are applied to the skin. Their chief characteristic is that they contain a very small amount of oil emulsified in a large amount of water, the significance of which I shall come to in a moment.

My first patient of the day arrives; she is tall and slim. I make a mental note of her appearance. She has long legs; she's obviously not wearing a bra and doesn't appear to need one. Her hair-do shows as little of her face as possible: fringe descending to the eyebrows, sides falling straight down to cover half the cheeks. What I can see of her face looks rather attractive, but it is plastered with make-up so thick you could cut it with a knife.

'Well, what can I do for you?' I ask.

'I've got this oily skin I can't seem to get rid of. I only did my face an hour ago, so it doesn't show yet, but in an hour or two my make-up will be completely shiny … '

' … and all patchy. I know. But in an hour's time you won't be here and I shan't be able to see it. You shouldn't have put on make-up before coming to see me. It's your skin I want to see, not the stuff you plaster on top of it. And even if I get you to remove your make-up now, I still won't be able to see anything because you'll de-grease your skin as you clean it. It's no good your telling me that you've got an oily skin; I need to see *how* oily it is, because mild seborrhea doesn't call for the same treatment as bad seborrhea.'

'Mine's bad all right.'

'I want to see that for myself. You're like those people who come to consult me about their greasy hair and give it a good shampooing the night before. Nothing looks more like a normal scalp than one which has just been shampooed, even if it is seborrheic. I tell them to come back four or five days after their last shampoo – often what they regard as an appalling case of seborrhea is no more than a mild one. Because they perspire a lot on the scalp, their hair goes damp and straggly as though it was very greasy. It's easy to confuse the two states unless you look very closely. And it's important not to make a mistake, because the treatment isn't the same ... What about you, do you have greasy hair, would you say? Remember that you can have seborrhea, even bad seborrhea, on the face without having it on the scalp as well. The two sometimes go together, but not necessarily.'

'No, I don't think my hair's greasy, apart from my fringe.'

'That's because of the seborrhea on your forehead. A fringe is a bad idea when the skin underneath it is oily. It makes you hot so that you sweat more than usual, and sweat spreads the seborrhea. It's a vicious circle.'

'Do you mean I should get rid of my fringe?'

'We'll see. First I must see you without make-up. We'll ignore this consultation and make another appointment.'

I saw her again shortly afterwards. She did indeed have very bad seborrhea and an extremely muddy-looking complexion. With a woebegone expression she allowed me to see the worst.

'Now you see why I have to plaster myself with stuff, as you put it.'

'Not at all, but we'll come to that in a minute. Tell me, how do you look after your skin? What do you use on your face last thing at night, for instance?'

'Soap and water.'

'What kind of soap?'

'I did try acid soaps, but they made my face smart.'

'I'm not surprised; they're harsh detergents which not only drastically de-grease the skin but also attack the chemical structure of the horny cells on the surface. These chemicals have an important protective role which we call the "barrier function"; for example, if the skin comes into contact with an alkaline substance such as soda, the acid in these chemicals will neutralise it. If they're weakened, the skin loses an important means of defence. Plain white soaps are the least harmful on the whole, but for years now I've banned the use of soap on the face, of whatever brand, and acid soaps above all. What do you use next?'

'I use a skin-tonic and then put on a camphorated cream for oily skin.'

'Does the tonic contain alcohol?'

'Yes.'

'And in the morning, what do you do?'

'I use a cleansing milk, wipe it off with the tonic, put on my tinted foundation and then powder over it. But I constantly have to re-powder my face; by the end of the day it looks awful; some days, I even have to renew my make-up completely once if not twice.'

'What's your job?'

'I'm a receptionist. I need to look presentable, but no matter what I do, it just gets worse.'

'I can quite believe it. You're doing everything possible to make it worse.'

I explain the phenomenon of reactive seborrhea.

'Now you can see why using a tonic based on alcohol and washing your face with soap won't do any good. But your tinted foundation may be doing even more harm.'

'If that means I have to stop using it, what on earth shall I do? I can't go around without make-up!'

All women protest violently if it's suggested that they stop using their foundation.

'Do you prefer to have a face which looks like a slab of buttered bread? Supposing I told you that your tinted foundation may well be the cause of your continuing seborrhea, would you still go on using it?'

'I don't see how my foundation can turn my skin oily.'

'Because what it does is to de-grease the skin. Let me explain it in this way: as you know, oil and water don't mix; if you pour olive oil into a saucer of water it forms globules on the surface. When you beat the mixture energetically, the oil disperses into tiny droplets, as it does if you're making a mayonnaise. Because it has disappeared, you think you've mixed it with the water, but, being lighter than water, it will rise to the surface again almost immediately, when the globules will reform.

'Nowadays there are special processes whereby cosmetic manufacturers can obtain homogenised, stable products from oils and water. These products are called "emulsions" and the substance used in making them, "emulsifiers"; of course, an emulsion isn't a solution of oil and water, because fats won't dissolve in water, but a suspension of minute particles of oil and minute particles of water, for which the emulsifier acts as a bond.

'This suspension can be obtained in two different ways: either by dispersing a small amount of oil – known as the oily phase – in a large amount of water – known as the aqueous phase – or inversely, by dispersing a small amount of water in a large amount of oil. In the first instance you get an oil-in-water emulsion, in the second, a water-in-oil emulsion.

'In manufacturing these emulsions, we're only imitating nature; without knowing it, you've been using natural emulsions since the day you were born: milk is a natural oil-in-water emulsion, and butter a water-in-oil emulsion. All modern cosmetics, creams and milks, are emulsions of one type or the other.

'Oil-in-water emulsions are the most widely used. Their popularity is largely due to their being so easy and pleasant to use: they don't appear to make the skin greasy because they contain only a small amount of oil, whereas the relatively large amount of water they contain gives an agreeable sensation of freshness as it evaporates. But for people with seborrhea, their pleasantness is more than outweighed by their drawbacks. Oil-in-water emulsions have the property of emulsifying the fats on the surface of the skin, in other words, they absorb them. The result is a de-greasing of the skin. In the same way, your tinted foundation aggravates the reactive seborrhea which you've already triggered off by using soap and alcohol-based tonic. So you mustn't be surprised if your face is flooded with sebum after an hour or two and glistens like a well-tossed salad: you're pumping out non-stop the secretion of your over-worked sebaceous glands.'

'How can I stop it happening?'

'By doing the opposite of everything you're doing now.

'I've even been known to give my patients two prescriptions. One goes as follows:

'To maintain or aggravate seborrhea:

1 Wash morning and night with soap, preferably acid;

2 Rub energetically with a 90° proof alcohol solution: it should be pure or camphorated or, best of all, contain tincture of iodine;

3 Apply a preparation containing sulphur;

4 Expose the face for long periods to the sun or, failing that, a sun-lamp;

5 Apply vanishing creams (oil-in-water emulsions) and especially foundation creams.

'The combination of these methods will greatly improve the chances of obtaining a highly satisfactory deterioration ... '

'But that's more or less what I've been doing for years, except for the sulphur which I gave up after one try because it made my skin so sore.'

'And just look at the result. It's just as well you didn't persevere with the sulphur.

'A year ago I happened to read, in one of the world's leading dermatological reviews, published in England, an account of a fascinating study carried out by Albert M. Kligman, an American Professor of Dermatology, in my view one of the most brilliant specialists in my field. Kligman is a man who advances the frontiers of knowledge because he challenges dogma, and he took a fresh look at the doctrine which states that sulphur is the treatment-par-excellence for acne. He actually had the temerity to question the use of sulphur, as sacred to dermatologists as cows to starving Indians; sulphur, contained in three-quarters of the creams, lotions and ointments sold over the counter in every self-respecting chemist's shop as remedies for acne; sulphur, which is "good for acne". Good for acne it unquestionably is! If acne could talk, it would say how delighted it was with these products which give it a new lease of life every time they are used. But it isn't good for the acne sufferer whose blackheads it helps to establish and increase.

'I've been making war on these preparations since 1954, because I know from clinical observations that they are not only ineffective but positively harmful. I published my conclusions and was abused for my pains. By pointing the finger at sulphur, I had broken a taboo! Kligman was able to do what I lacked the opportunity of doing: American resources are more powerful than ours. He made

a scientific study of the effects of sulphur on the sebaceous glands
of both laboratory animals and human volunteers.

'Kligman was able to demonstrate once and for all that sulphur
is comedogenic, in other words, that it causes the formation of
blackheads in men and animals. You don't have to be an expert to
see the absurdity of treating a disease whose primary lesion is the
blackhead by applying a product which actually encourages its
formation. One might as well try to put out a fire by pouring on
oil!'

'Why did you say just now that you couldn't carry out these
experiments yourself?'

'Quite simply, I lacked the necessary "guinea-pigs".'

A SHORT DIGRESSION ON CLINICAL TESTS
WITH THE HELP OF VOLUNTEERS

It should be emphasised that clinical tests of this sort are neither
dangerous nor painful for the human 'guinea-pigs' involved:
before applying the substance to be tested, a small piece of skin is
removed; this process, known as a 'biopsy', is then repeated after
the product has been applied regularly for some weeks. The biopsies are done under anaesthetic, a local one, of course, and you
don't feel a thing. The skin fragment itself is no more than five or
six millimetres in diameter. One or two stitches of nylon thread
are sufficient to close the incision and they leave no visible trace,
especially if the site chosen is in a natural fold of the skin.

Some people still dislike the idea of tests being carried out on
human beings. They are essential to progress nevertheless, for tests
on animals can only give us a general indication; they can tell us
whether or not a new drug is dangerous, for example, which is the
main thing; but apart from this, you can't know for certain until
you try whether a particular reaction observed in rats, mice,
rabbits or dogs will be exactly reproduced in human beings. Tests
like these therefore have an enormous collective and scientific
value, as well as being devoid of risk for those willing to take part
in them.

I've only had the chance to carry out similar tests three times
in my whole career: on the first occasion, my object was to verify
the innocuousness of a product which browns the skin artificially.
The volunteers came from the manufacturer's laboratory and

knew that their product was harmless in principle. Having examined skin biopsies taken before and after ten days of repeated applications, I was able to confirm this. There was no ensuing irritation, not even on the eyelids, the most delicate area of the skin.

On the second occasion, which I shall describe in a later chapter, I was concerned with embryonic extracts.

My object on the third occasion was to discover whether, in human beings, creams of the oil-in-water variety provoked the same extraordinary and quite unexpected reaction as the one I had accidentally found in real guinea-pigs: one very often stumbles on new facts by chance.

When this type of cream is applied to the skin of guinea-pigs the sebaceous glands are seen to enlarge and triple or even quadruple in volume.

Now in people with oily skins, one of the characteristics of the sebaceous glands is that they are much larger than normal.

It was a significant point; I had long suspected that certain cosmetics were making my patients' skin oily, without being able to explain how or why. If I could reproduce the same effect on human skin, I would have my answer: this time it wasn't so much a question of the de-greasing effect produced by these preparations, which trigger bouts of reactive seborrhea through the mechanism I have described, but of a possible direct stimulation of the sebaceous glands as well. And this was exactly what the clinical test enabled me to confirm: while the effect of oil-in-water emulsions on human sebaceous glands is not so spectacular as on the sebaceous glands of animals, it undoubtedly exists. So you can see why I always forbid any patient of mine to use any cosmetic which falls into that category.

I was able to find six volunteers to help me in my demonstration: a medical student, a young chemist and four nuns who saw a chance to earn a little money for charity – I feel it's only right to compensate people who agree to take part in such tests. It's not a question of compensation in the legal sense, the price of pain, since no pain is involved; it's some remuneration for the volunteers' collaboration, their time and the various tasks they must carry out faithfully for the duration of the experiment: in this case applying a given amount of the preparation to a particular area regularly night and morning for six weeks and turning up punctually on eight separate occasions—four times for the biopsies to be performed and four times for the stitches to be removed; even when it's a question of purely scientific, non-profit-making research, such as this was, it wouldn't occur to me to ask people to put up with all that inconvenience for nothing. Of course, if people are prepared to do it for love, one can only respect them the more for it.

In any case, an allowance is always made in the budget for fees to the participants in these experiments.* I use the word fees deliberately because, while the experiment is going on, the volunteer is the doctor's colleague, co-operating with him in the interests of science or the community; of science when it's a question of disinterested research, of the community when financial interests are involved.

ALLERGY TESTS

Patch tests for allergy are a typical example of what I mean. As you may know, all chemical substances, without exception, can cause allergic reactions which are manifested as eczema. This form of eczema is known as 'contact eczema' because it results from external contact. (It's also called 'contact dermatitis', which is the same thing.)

The substance which causes the allergy is called an 'allergen'. Any product, whether vegetable or mineral, a cosmetic or an item of clothing, whether used during medical treatment or at work, may be responsible. There are strong allergens, which cause eczema in a great many people, and weak allergens, which can be used with the minimum of risk; there are also hypo-allergens, which are, practically speaking, harmless. *But in terms of allergic response no substance is completely harmless.*

Let's suppose that a chemist has discovered something which has possibilities in the cosmetic field. At the outset, no one knows whether it's a strong, weak or very weak allergen. It must first be tested. Tests are the only way of avoiding the possibility of an epidemic of contact dermatitis once a product is on the market and its use unsupervised and unrestricted.

We therefore do what are called 'patch tests' on volunteers by applying the product to the skin over a period of forty-eight hours.

* In 1976 this practice applied on occasion in the U.S.A. but not usually in the United Kingdom. (Tr)

All that needs to be done is to impregnate a small piece of gauze about a centimetre square with the substance to be tested, often diluted, and keep it in place with sticking-plaster. If there's a positive reaction the worst that can happen is that there'll be a little redness accompanied by slight itching; this is restricted to the point of application and passes off within a day or two.

When a patient already has eczema, we always do a patch test to identify the precise cause of his rash; until the cause has been identified it can't be eliminated, and until it is eliminated the eczema will persist. Supposing you were to develop eczema and your nail-varnish was suspected, there's only one way you could be cured: first you would have to have patch tests to prove that it was your nail-varnish which was responsible, then you must never use it again.

But surely, you may object, the first tests I mentioned are different, because the volunteers don't have eczema.

That is true, of course, but there's no fundamental difference; the test we make in order to pinpoint the cause of an existing eczema are diagnostic tests, whereas those we make in order to discover the degree to which a new product is allergenic are called 'prophetic' tests. In the United States a manufacturer wishing to market a new dermatological or cosmetic preparation is obliged by law to carry out these tests in order to protect the public from un-expected or unpleasant side-effects; that's what I meant just now when I talked of the interests of the community.

Even where they're not obligatory, as in France, they're still practised as a matter of course; it's in a manufacturer's own interest to avoid the distribution of products which, if they were to cause an epidemic, would do considerable harm to his brand image.

THE RIGHT WAY TO TREAT AN OILY SKIN

But to get back to the subject of my patient's seborrhea.

'I'm going to ask you', I assured her, 'to stop using all those methods of treatment which, however slightly, are helping to main-tain your condition – if not actually making it worse.

'The kind of mild seborrhea which drags on interminably is very common, simply because it is wrongly or unsuitably treated: only give it the proper care, and it'll soon clear up. Be kind to your skin and it'll return the compliment. Of course, when I say skin I include your scalp and your hair.

'I know of nothing more misleading than so-called "medicated" shampoos labelled "for oily hair".

'As though a shampoo could possibly be a medicine! It's nothing more than liquid soap. Do you believe that you're "treating" your skin when you have a bath or a shower with your favourite soap? —you're getting rid of the dirt, nothing more. And it's to be hoped that your soap is a good quality one, without too much detergent in it. A good soap should contain the bare minimum of detergent, just enough to remove the deposits and impurities which cling to the surface of the skin without attacking the skin itself. If your skin needs treatment it certainly won't get it from your soap.

'Equally the most you can expect from a shampoo is that it will clean your hair without harming it, and, if you have oily hair, that it won't de-grease the scalp so drastically that you're caught in the vicious circle of reactive seborrhea.

'Liquid or solid, it's the quality of the soap which counts; soft soap, which contains caustic potash, is a notorious irritant; plain white soaps which contain soda are much less harmful, as long as they're well "salted out", to use manufacturers' jargon; that is, with no crude alkali left in them to irritate the skin as there is in cheap soaps.

'It's less well-known that mass-produced shampoos and the acid liquid soaps which some people use instead are made from detergents not dissimilar to industrial detergents. If it's clean hair you want, they'll clean it—with brutal thoroughness. Your hair and face shouldn't be scoured like your pots and pans.

'Don't expect a soap or a shampoo to do the impossible, to treat your skin or hair; the most you can hope for is that they won't do your condition any positive harm, which shouldn't be too much to ask. In any case, how could they "treat" your skin when they're only in contact with it for a few brief moments? Speaking for myself, I only wish I knew the treatment capable of acting in two minutes. Even powerfully acting preparations, such as ointments containing cortisone derivatives, take up to three days to calm a skin inflammation at the best of times. It's obvious from this alone that no shampoo has the ability to treat. On the other hand, a harsh detergent can harm your hair in no time. All that one demands of such preparations is that they should be neutral. And as long as manufacturers continue to insist on marketing shampoos for oily, dry and normal hair according to ideas that are fifty years out of date, I shall continue to advise patients with oily hair to use only those shampoos for dry or brittle hair.

'I take the precaution of warning them that I haven't taken leave of my senses, that I'm perfectly responsible for my actions in advising them to use this type of shampoo, so that when they get home and read the label they don't rush to the telephone and ask my secretary if I'm feeling all right, or if she's noticed me behaving strangely of late!

'I'm relatively happy about these shampoos, especially when they contain substances called "lipo-proteins" which are the least likely to cause reactive seborrhea. I even advise boys with seborrhea to use some brands on their faces.'

'But not girls?'

'No, because their skin isn't as tough as boys'. Girls should only use cleansing milks. The same thing is true of boys with fair hair and very sensitive skin: I get them to use a cleansing milk too.'

'What sort of cleansing milk?'

'It doesn't matter as long as it's not one of the brands which contain detergent, "astringent", or "skin-toner". Again, neutrality is the guide-line.'

'But I never feel my skin's really clean after I've used a cleansing milk.'

'That's just an idea you've got into your head. A cleansing milk is every bit as effective as soap, as long as you use it properly. Cleansing milk is an oil-in-water emulsion containing plenty of water. This type of preparation cleans by emulsifying impurities soluble in water in its aqueous phase and impurities soluble in oil in its oily phase. Consequently it cleans very thoroughly provided that you don't put it on with cotton-wool. The best thing to do is to rub it in with your hands, as you do when you soap your face, then wipe it off carefully with a dry tissue before rinsing; never leave the smallest trace of cleansing milk on your skin, firstly because, as I've just explained, being an oil-in-water emulsion it can cause bouts of reactive seborrhea, and secondly because your skin won't be clean; you'd be surprised how many women deliberately leave a little cleansing milk on their skin in order, as they put it, to "nourish" it, not realising that what they are leaving behind as "nourishment" for their precious skin is a mixture of milk and dirt. Hardly the ideal skin-food! Most of the milk will be removed by wiping and rinsing will do the rest. You can use cotton-wool; damp cotton-wool won't irritate the skin.'

'What should I rinse with?'

'Just water; if the tap-water is very hard you should use distilled water, or else, if you want to be sophisticated about it, one of those preparations pompously labelled "tonics" — but it must be alcohol-free.

'Why they're called "tonics" I can't imagine. A tonic is something which fortifies and invigorates. In order to fortify a skin, an ingredient would first have to penetrate it and, clearly, a tonic can no more penetrate the skin than water can. Nevertheless, most women manage to turn it into yet another method of damaging their skin. Tell me, do you dry your face with a tissue after using your tonic?'

'No, I leave it to dry.'

'Like nine women out of ten. Have you thought what would happen if every time you washed your hands, you omitted to dry them properly? I'll tell you: after two or three days they would be so chapped you wouldn't be able to bend your fingers.

'What makes you think the skin on your face is any different? In the case of someone with very bad seborrhea it doesn't matter so much, but for people with normal skin, and especially for those with dried-up skin, it's a disastrous habit. You should always dry your skin when it's damp.

'To sum up, you should use a cleansing milk on your face at night, scrupulously removing every trace, and carefully wiping it dry after rinsing. In the morning, all you need do is to rinse with clean water or a neutral lotion, making sure once more that you dry carefully afterwards.'

'Then can I make up?'

(This is the main worry of all my women patients and one can't blame them; they need to mask their imperfections at all costs, and they're afraid lest I should be so insensitive as to ban all make-up for medical reasons: hadn't I just pounced on the mere mention of foundation creams?)

'You can make up, but not in your usual way. I'm going to suggest that you use a cream which is the opposite of the one you've been using — a water-in-oil emulsion.* Emulsions of this type

* See footnote on p. 78. (Tr)

are rich in oil. You may be surprised at my suggesting that you use an oily cream on an oily skin, but in fact it's the only way to help stabilise your seborrhea. Unlike oil-in-water emulsions – which, as I told you, tripled or even quintupled the volume of sebaceous glands in laboratory animals – water-in-oil emulsions don't affect the size of the sebaceous glands, or if they do, it's to reduce them. Water-in-oil emulsions thus have a genuinely stabilising effect. When you spread this type of cream over the skin it mixes with the natural fats and so avoids de-greasing the epidermal surface. Consequently, this cream entails no risk of reactive seborrhea. And, up to a point, the flow of sebum is stemmed. It should be used very sparingly, and it takes time to learn how much to put on; to begin with you may have to wipe off any excess with a tissue.'

'Do I only use it in the mornings?'

'If you had mild seborrhea, that would be sufficient. In the case of bad seborrhea like yours, however, when what is required is a sustained effect, you need to use it night and morning.'

'What do I put on top of it, as you say I mustn't use foundation?'

'Just face-powder.'

'But that's out of the question! What on earth would I look like?'

I've been expecting this reaction and greet it unmoved.

'You'll certainly look better than you do when your foundation is glistening with sebum! If I were to be unkind, I'd say that you couldn't look worse. You've got nothing to lose by trying out my suggestion.'

'It looks as though I've no choice!'

'Alas, you have, but I think you'd be making a great mistake if you persisted in your old ways, now that you know the consequences. A beauty-product that is harmful to the skin is quite indefensible, no matter how convenient it may be to use. Once you've learnt how to powder over the cream, I assure you that you won't need any more convincing.'

'What do I do?'

'There's a well-tried method that seems to have been forgotten in these days of foundation creams; it consists of putting on twice as much powder as you normally use over the cream base, then dampening it – with a spray, if you like. Next you pat it in, without rubbing, with a tissue. In this way, the particles of damp powder are pressed into the film of cream. The excess of powder gives you an all-over, matt effect which will last, won't go patchy and, providing that you've chosen a colour to harmonise with your complexion, will look more natural than any other form of make-up. It's a knack; it may take you a couple of minutes longer than putting on your foundation cream, but your patience will be rewarded.'

'Just now, when you were talking about the various ways of aggravating seborrhea, you mentioned the sun. I'm going skiing in a couple of weeks and I've no intention of spending my holiday shut up in an hotel!'

'I'm not such a tyrant as that! However, you must give your face the maximum protection with a sun-screen — *not* sun-tan — preparation. And that means applying it several times a day. The protective film which you put on your face at nine in the morning won't even last you until eleven o'clock, and the most dangerous time of day is between eleven and two o'clock in the afternoon.'

'So my face won't get brown?'

'The less you tan, the happier I shall be. Among its other harmful properties, the sun — or to be more precise, its ultra-violet rays — has the effect of thickening the horny layer of epidermis.

'In people with seborrhea whose pores are open, this can cause the formation of tiny horny plugs which prevent the sebum from flowing freely over the epidermis; instead it accumulates to form closed comedones, making the skin look lumpy. So, you see, the sun can turn a simple case of seborrhea into acne.

'As for those people who already have acne, together with the horny thickening which blocks the pores, they will be made irretrievably worse.

'It's a myth that sunlight is good for acne. People think it must be beneficial because they see their spots dry up due to the antiseptic effect of the ultra-violet rays. Furthermore, when you have a tan, blackheads and acne scars don't show up so much. You have the illusion of an improvement, whereas what is really happening is that you're building up a stock of closed comedones which will develop into appalling acne within three or four weeks.

'The two months after his return from holiday are the worse months of the year for the acne sufferer. Of course there's no such thing as an absolute, universal rule in medicine. The secondary effects I've just described aren't always so dramatic. However they are frequent enough for me to consider acne patients cured only when they can expose themselves to the sun, within reason, without a relapse.

E

'Personally, preferring prevention to cure, I err deliberately on the side of caution when patients ask me for advice: I would rather they didn't take the risk. All the effort and achievement that have gone into a year's treatment can be ruined by a month's carelessness.'

SEBORRHEA AND THE PILL

'And is that all I need do to get rid of my seborrhea?'

'Far from it. If you only had mild seborrhea I would say yes. But where it's acute, as in your case, local applications to the skin do no more than keep it under control. You can only be cured by treatment from within.'

'Do you mean I should go on a diet?'

'No. With seborrhea, as with acne, dieting has no effect whatever. A disease whose origins are hormonal can't be cured by restricting what you eat. Your treatment has to act on the endocrine system, and that means using hormones. These days, the best hormonal treatment for women with seborrhea and acne is the contraceptive pill.'

'But I've been on the pill for a year and it hasn't done any good.'

'What kind are you taking?'

She named two different brands which she had tried in succession.

'In that case, I'm not surprised they had no effect! All types of the pill may act as contraceptives, but, from the dermatological point of view, some are very different from others. Tell me, do you know what's in the pill?'

'Not really, no.'

'In principle, the pill combines the action of two of the hormones secreted by the ovaries: the female hormone, oestrogen, and the hormone which prepares the uterus for possible pregnancy every month, progesterone. In practice, instead of natural hormones, synthetic agents are used whose chemical structure closely resembles them and which possess exactly the same properties.

'The amount of oestrogen varies from one brand of pill to another: some contain 100 micrograms, others 80, others 75, and some only 50. The latter are what we call 'mini-pills'. In the case of the second hormone, represented by 'progesterones' (all of which, of course, possess the properties of progesterone), there is one very significant fact: *certain progesterones also possess properties similar to those of the male hormone.*

'I myself have helped to demonstrate that any brand of the pill which contains less than 80 thousandths of a milligram of oestrogen is totally inactive in acne. That's why the mini-pill you've been taking for the past year has been ineffective. It contains sufficient oestrogen to prevent an unwanted pregnancy, but not enough to get rid of your seborrhea.

'In dealing with seborrhea and acne we can divide the various brands of the pill into two categories: those which have a curative effect and those which have no effect at all.

'However, there's also a third category: those which have an aggravating effect. It was lucky for you that you weren't given one of them, for they're very commonly prescribed. They are the brands in which the progesterones possess properties analogous to those of the male hormone; for someone like you, whose sebaceous glands are abnormally sensitive to the male hormone, they would have had extremely unfortunate consequences. Ordinarily they can be taken without ill-effect, but a person with seborrhea mustn't touch them.

'I'm going to prescribe a brand of the pill for you which contains a harmless derivative of progesterone together with the amount of female hormone necessary to have a beneficial effect on your seborrhea; that is, 100 thousandths of a milligram. As brands go, it's considered to be "strong", because it contains twice as much oestrogen as is needed to prevent contraception. I shall therefore ask you to take certain precautions – which you ought to observe in any case, with whatever brand of the pill, even the weakest. In this way, you'll run no risks, and, within four to six months, you'll no longer have that shiny face. I hasten to say that I can't promise the same in the case of your hair. It might show an equal improvement, but one can't be certain. We still don't know why, in the same person, the pill doesn't automatically have the same effect on seborrhea of the scalp as it has on seborrhea of the face.'

FRENCHWOMEN AND THE PILL

Only about two million Frenchwomen take the pill, in other words, a small minority. It is strikingly few, considering that there are about ten million women of childbearing age in France. In some cases, this resistance to the pill can be explained by religious factors, but where the remainder are concerned it seems to be essentially linked either to a complete lack of information or to misleading information spread by word of mouth, with the result that there's a climate of suspicion, if not panic, surrounding these drugs, for all the world as though they were imbued with some mysterious power or supernatural evil.

At a time when it's fashionable to talk about things being 'natural' or otherwise, most people are surprised to learn that the pill is natural, in that it's a facsimile of the hormones which circulate in the blood and are indispensable to their health and well-being. Moreover, where the effects of the pill are concerned, the absorption of these hormones merely subdues certain natural phenomena without tampering with them: the best proof of this is that the changes wrought by them are reversible.

I have prescribed the pill for women suffering from seborrhea and acne for many years now, and during that time I've heard some remarks that are almost unbelievable.

Ignorance has always been the Establishment's best weapon for keeping the public quiet. Ignorance prevents people from making up their own minds, choosing or criticising. By concealing the true facts surrounding a problem, it's easy to mislead people about the intentions and motives underlying decisions which affect them and to ensure their compliance. What have the French authorities done until now to enlighten the public about the facts of contraception? Absolutely nothing.

It took fifteen years of sustained effort before a small group of doctors in France managed to bring about the repeal of a law that, by forbidding the dissemination of information about methods of contraception as well as contraceptives themselves, reduced women to the status of objects, fifteen years before a new law was passed permitting the use of contraceptives and recognising women as individuals in their own right.

Enlightened attitudes can hardly be expected to flourish in an atmosphere of equivocation, false ideas, obscurantism and lies. Handing over a prescription for the pill is quite unlike handing over a prescription for any other medicine; each time, you must allay anxieties, explain, correct misapprehensions.

'The trouble with the pill,' I'm told, 'is that we don't really understand it.'

But of course we do. Contraceptive pills are made from hormones that were known and employed in medicine long before the pill was invented. What's new about them isn't the hormones they contain, but the way in which these hormones are used. We use them to inhibit the function of the ovaries, thus rendering a woman sterile for as long as she continues to take them.

But the pill isn't only a contraceptive; it can also be remarkably effective in treating a number of gynaecological disorders: menstrual pains, for example, or cases where the ovary secretes an abnormal amount of male hormone, or even endometriosis,* a disease previously curable only by surgery and then, alas, not always successfully.

– 'The pill is dangerous!'

Any active drug can be dangerous precisely because it's active. Even a common drug like penicillin can cause appalling mishaps. And common or garden aspirin is responsible for many more disasters than the pill. Every year, in England, twenty-nine young children die because aspirin has been carelessly administered; aspirin can cause intestinal haemorrhages and acute urticaria which, when it affects the throat, can obstruct breathing if not caught in time.

The administration of any drug is bound by rules which must be scrupulously observed. What women must never do is to choose a brand of pill 'off the peg', as it were, without taking those precautions which reduce to a minimum such risks as there are – and these, being relatively few and perfectly well-known, are easily avoidable.

The most serious is the risk of phlebitis and embolism: before embarking on a course of the pill, a blood-test for cholesterol and blood-fats must be done, and repeated at the end of the first, third and sixth course of treatment; each course lasts from twenty to twenty-two days depending on the brand of pill.

The pill should never be prescribed for women with bad leg veins, which is anyway uncommon at the age when you suffer from seborrhea; women on the pill with a history of phlebitis on their maternal side should be carefully watched; sufferers from true migraine shouldn't take the pill, or should stop taking it if it brings on an attack (but migraine, which is a quite distinct disease,

---

* A disease caused by small amounts of the lining of the womb spreading outside the uterine cavity. They cause acute pain during menstruation. (A-B)

shouldn't be confused with the common headache which accompanies a hangover, indigestion, a cold or 'flu).

– 'The pill makes you put on weight!'

All reliable statistics show that 60 per cent of women on the pill suffer no change in weight, 20 per cent lose weight and only 20 per cent put it on. An increase in weight due to the pill is thus far from inevitable. The minority who do gain weight fall into three main groups:

1 Those with a tendency to water-retention, especially during the pre-menstrual period;

2 Those with a predisposition to diabetes; that is, women who have a history of diabetes in the family. This hereditary factor doesn't mean that the descendants are or will be diabetic, it simply increases the risk of their being so. In this case, the pill acts as a discloser of trouble which would be revealed in the course of any hormonal treatment. A gain in weight of more than three kilograms in a woman who is on the pill is an indication for a test for blood-sugar. From one point of view this is a good, rather than a bad thing: such patients are bound to become diabetic in the long run; the disease usually comes to light around the age of forty, after having evolved unnoticed for some time during which it will have caused severe damage in a variety of ways, especially to the arteries. The early discovery of this predisposition, this threat, thanks to the pill, allows preventive measures to be taken and the disease to be caught in time.

3 A gain in weight in women on the pill only rarely signifies diabetes, however; more often than not it turns out to be the result of immoderate or obsessive eating. Of the 20 per cent of women who put on weight, the majority are either greedy or frustrated; the former gorge themselves while assuring you that they hardly eat a thing, and are most indignant when you accuse them of over-eating; the latter seek refuge in food: with each mouthful they are compensating for their lack of sexual, emotional or professional satisfaction; they spend their time raiding the refrigerator to appease a sense of continual hunger. They don't eat much at a time, but they're always nibbling at something. Not surprisingly, both types of women find the pill an excellent scapegoat for their gain in weight. The plain fact is that, except in rare cases of water-

retention or diabetes, nobody puts on weight unless he eats too much; if you save more than you spend, you increase your capital. In this case, the capital is fat. It's true that the pill increases the appetite — but if you keep a watch on it, there's no need to put on weight. The pill by itself doesn't cause overweight.

— 'The pill causes cancer!'

It has now been proved that cancer of the uterus is more common in women who don't take the pill than in those who do; it therefore appears that the pill gives some form of protection against this type of cancer.

As far as cancer of the breast is concerned, claims have been made for both good and bad effects of the pill, and numerous studies have failed to clarify the situation. A few years ago, in America, public opinion was stirred up by experiments made on beagles. The dogs were given the pill and developed breast tumours. Nobody bothered to point out that this particular breed of dog is subject to spontaneous tumours and, more often than not, breast tumours; not only that, they were given the pill in very large doses, much larger than those prescribed for women. Finally, the tumours developed by the beagles turned out to be benign, as dogs' tumours normally are, and not cancerous.

You don't have to be a scientist to realise that these experiments proved nothing at all. A great deal of fuss surrounded the story nevertheless, because anything to do with the pill is an excuse for sensationalism.

The truth is that no one is certain of the facts; women who have been treated for breast-cancer have taken the pill without suffering a recurrence. As yet, there's not the slightest evidence that the pill can cause breast-cancer, but until we know more about it, to be on the safe side we prefer not to prescribe the pill for women with cysts of the breast in order to avoid any risk of encouraging the natural tendency of such cysts to become cancerous.

— 'Women on the pill risk having deformed babies!'

This notion was the subject of a detailed study carried out in France. The investigators' conclusions were unequivocal: the frequency of foetal malformations is no greater among those women who take the pill than those who don't; and where there is a malformation, it's so gross that the embryo is unviable and miscarriage inevitably follows.

A woman who has been on the pill therefore runs no greater risk of giving birth to a deformed baby than one who has never taken it.

In order to avoid the unpleasantness and disappointment of a miscarriage, it's advisable for women who stop taking the pill in order to conceive to take other precautions for a few weeks before starting a baby. Three months is sufficient: the average length of time required for the periods to return to normal—they will often be late on the first two or three occasions.

During this interval, simple means of protection such as the vaginal diaphragm, or a male contraceptive device, are better than trying to use the 'safe' period, when the best calculations are liable to go awry because of the irregularity of the periods.

—'There's a risk of multiple birth with the pill!'

There's no such risk whatsoever. It used to be thought that the pill was one method of treating sterility, but we know today that it is not. Certain types of sterility can be treated by quite different hormones which may, if not administered with the utmost care, stimulate the ovary to produce several ova at the same time.

—'The pill makes your hair fall out!'

It's true that certain brands of the pill can have such undesirable side-effects in people already so predisposed. The same brands are inclined to aggravate seborrhea. It's better to avoid using them if you have a slightly oily skin or a tendency to produce too much body-hair.

All other brands are harmless in this respect, and some of them, those that we use in the treatment of seborrhea and acne, can occasionally have a beneficial effect on hair-loss in women. In other words, it's quite wrong to generalise and say that the pill makes your hair fall out.

—'The pill encourages promiscuity among the young!'

That reminds me of a story. One of my closest friends, an intelligent, civilised, open-minded man, sent his daughter to see me; she had a nasty facial seborrhea which was ruining her looks. I had known her since she was a child. She was now grown-up and had developed into quite a strong, self-willed personality. Without thinking twice about it, I asked her, as I ask all my young female patients in order to gain an impression of the gynaecological and psychological background to their seborrhea:

'Are you still a virgin?'

She had complete confidence in me and our relationship was

absolutely relaxed. Without the slightest hesitation, perfectly naturally, she replied 'no'.

'How long have you been having sex?'

'For two years.'

'Do you use a contraceptive?'

'No!'

'And you haven't had ... a slip-up?'

'No.'

'Do you want to have a baby?'

'Oh! Certainly not! At any rate, not yet.'

'In that case, you're not only being extremely foolish but very lucky. Hasn't it occurred to you that if you make love you're liable to get pregnant?'

'Of course, but we take precautions.'

— The sort of precautions that, 40 per cent of the time, end in slip-ups and lead to between 600,000 and 800,000 back-street abortions every year in France alone, procured by probes, knitting-needles, parsley stalks or injections of soapy water, resulting in several deaths and many women being rendered sterile for life.

'Don't you realise that your precautions are hardly any better than leaving things to chance?'

'Yes, but I never think it'll happen to me.'

— They're all the same, these girls; other people get into trouble, never them — until it happens.

'Listen to me. You must do whatever you think best; it's your problem and not for me to judge; moralising isn't my job. But I wouldn't like anything to happen which would cause a family crisis, and despite your air of independence, a crisis in your life, too. Machiavelli said that love is sweet in the hearts of the young; but it's also, in its physical consummation, a responsible act. It's unforgivable to treat conceiving a baby like catching a cold. It should be a mutual, conscious decision; it must be deliberate. If you don't want to have a baby, you must act accordingly; not by having an abortion, but by taking proper precautions. If you want to live an adult life, you must behave like an adult. In order to treat your skin, I'm going to put you on the pill. At the same time, you'll no longer run the risk ... '

What had I done!

That same evening I received an agitated telephone call from her mother and then, a moment or two later, from her father.

'Robert, you've known her most of her life; she's very self-willed, she's had a lot of boy-friends and she's shown an interest in sex from an early age. If you put her on the pill, there'll be no holding her ... '

He didn't quite accuse me of leading his daughter astray, but he came close to it.

I tried to point out that young girls' morals were not dictated by the pill, that with or without it they would make love when they were ready to. It was no good. He made me promise to find some other method of treatment and I told him a white lie without the slightest remorse. There *was* no better way of treating her skin; moreover, I couldn't let her go on as she was without a proper contraceptive. I therefore continued surreptitiously to prescribe the pill for her until the day when her skin was cured and she married the man she loved.

When that day came, I violated professional secrecy with her consent and told her father everything. He was very sporting about it and I'm sure that I managed to change his ideas about the pill in relation to young girls for the better. In my opinion to make their virtue depend on such considerations is to put it at a very low level indeed.

The fact is that for years now I've been giving the pill to hundreds of young virgins with acne over long periods: the treatment must be continued for at least a year or eighteen months if the disappearance of the seborrhea or acne, usually achieved within four to six months, is to be lasting. There's always the likelihood of a relapse if, in the first flush of success, you're in too much of a hurry to stop the treatment.

Every one of these girls was quite well aware that she was benefiting from complete contraceptive protection throughout her treatment, yet those who lost their virginity over this period were very few indeed, and they told me quite openly that they would have done so in any case, and that the pill had played a very minor role in their decision. I haven't the slightest reason to doubt their word.

THE TREATMENT OF ACNE IN MEN

Where do men stand in all this?

When we talk of any skin trouble which affects the looks and how to deal with it, we usually think in terms of women, as though it didn't matter to men and there was no point in their worrying about it.

In fact, men worry about their skin almost as much as women. The only difference between the sexes is that boys begin to worry about it later than girls; but though a boy's awareness may be slower, it has equal repercussions on his psyche and behaviour, and deserves at least as much attention.

This is all the more true when you consider that in the case of seborrhea and acne, his disfigurement is usually the more serious and persistent of the two. It's also more common: seven out of every ten adolescent boys are affected. This male predominance where over-stimulation of the sebaceous apparatus is concerned is easily explicable: you only have to remember that the male hormone is responsible and that, obviously, a man will almost always secrete it in greater quantities than a woman. I say almost always because it can happen that in certain glandular diseases women secrete as much, or even more, than a normal man. In such cases, which are fortunately rare, female seborrhea can be as bad as the worst male seborrhea; but as a general rule it's the boy who is the unenviable winner in this competition. And he doesn't even have make-up to fall back on in order to camouflage his blemishes, any more than he does the pill. Not that the pill wouldn't have the same effect on him, dermatologically speaking as it does on his girl-friend: his seborrhea would clear up, his complexion cease to look muddy and return to normal, his skin become less coarse; but at the same time he would find himself developing certain pleasing curves on the chest as, inversely, his genital organs shrank and he became totally indifferent to the most expert sexual advances. It can readily be imagined that the few trials that were attempted in America elicited no enthusiasm whatever — not many men were prepared to pay the price of their virility for the disappearance of their acne!

So far, where the male sex is concerned, no hormone administered internally has proved to be completely satisfactory and without undesirable side-effects.

Research is currently going on to find preparations that can be applied to the diseased areas of the skin but which, being retained in those areas, don't have systemic, or more widespread, internal effects. The object of these experiments is to find a product which will compete with the male hormone on its own ground, that is, in the sebaceous glands, and so prevent it from exercising its stimulating properties.

Various avenues have been explored: those involving substances derived from the female hormone, and those involving substances which have the property of being anti-androgenic, that is, anti-male hormone. Interesting and encouraging research results are already emerging; but the percentage of success so far is lower than that obtained by means of the pill in women, who are still luckier than men in this respect.

This doesn't mean that men should think that they're the pariahs of oily skin, that they must live with their seborrhea, and that nothing can be done for them.

There are certain antibiotics that, when given in small doses over long periods, will help calm down their spots. More often than not, however, I find that these long-drawn-out courses of antibiotics are the source of anxiety to the patient, or to his mother, wife, sister or family friend. One immediately senses reservations which they don't like to put into words; but they are easily anticipated because, where antibiotics are concerned, the same two anxieties always lurk unspoken in the background: antibiotics have a debilitating effect on people, and people become resistant to them.

'Are you afraid that the antibiotics will make you run down?' I ask him.

'Yes, you see I'm about to take my exams ... '

And often his parent will elaborate:

'He's a bit run down as it is, and the last time he had a sore throat the doctor gave him penicillin because he was running a high temperature; it was weeks before he felt himself again.'

'It didn't occur to you that it was the sore throat and the high temperature that left him feeling weak?'

'No.'

'Nevertheless, that's the reason. Antibiotics are not debilitating in themselves; it's the illness which they're designed to combat which leaves you feeling under the weather. If my colleague had allowed the infection to run its course without antibiotics, this young man would have felt just the same, if not worse, because it would have lasted much longer.

'Don't forget that whereas an acute infection requires large doses of antibiotics, much smaller doses are sufficient for acne.'

'Even with big deep-seated spots like the ones on his neck?'

'Even with spots like his, for they're really more of an inflammation – the skin's reaction, if you like, to the irritant foreign body, the newly-formed closed comedone – than an infection. If you were to analyse the pus they contain, you would find ordinary non-virulent microbes – quite different from those found in a boil, for example, where the germ responsible is an extremely virulent one.

'As you know, you can be vaccinated against boils, but the same vaccine is ineffective in acne because the spots, however big and deep-seated, are not the same as boils.'

'That's right: he was vaccinated against boils and while he was having the injections he seemed a little better, but then the spots started all over again.'

'Exactly. The antibiotics used in acne act quite differently: they inhibit the special microbes found in all blackheads, microbes which manufacture an enzyme. This enzyme transforms certain fatty elements into what are called fatty acids. And it's the fatty acids which irritate and inflame the skin. By neutralising the activity of these microbes you prevent the transformation of the fat into fatty acids and stop the inflammation.'

'But the doctor tried giving him antibiotics twice last year and they didn't work.'

'Which antibiotics?'

'Well ... one of them was an ointment.'

'What was it called?'

There's always a long silence at this point. It's very rare for a patient to remember what medicaments he has been given. Much remains to be done to educate people in this respect: it can be extremely important, especially with a chronic ailment, to know the results, the success or failure, of a previous treatment. This knowledge can be significant in a number of ways, and people should always keep a note of any drugs they have taken. I try to help him.

'Did the name have "neomycin" in it?'

'That's right.'

'By itself?'

'No, I think there was something else as well.'

I suggest the name of a preparation combining a derivative of hydrocortisone with neomycin.

'That's it.'

'In that case, I can't say I'm surprised that it didn't work. Neomycin is an antibiotic which has no effect whatsoever on the germ which causes acne; and the other ingredient encourages the formation of keratin plugs that block the pores and is consequently more than likely to make the acne worse; cases have even been known where it has been the sole cause of a special form of acne known as "corticosteroid" acne. A product of this type should therefore never be used on a seborrheic skin. But didn't you mention a second treatment?'

'Yes, he was given antibiotics by mouth.'

'For how long did he take them?'

'About eight to ten days.'

'What sort of dose, how many capsules a day?'

'Six or eight; no, eight to begin with, then six.'

'That was both far too short a time and far too large a dose. Even those antibiotics which are most effective in acne only begin to work after a couple of weeks; that's why, for acne, they must be taken over long periods. And because they act by accumulating in the sebaceous glands, it's pointless to give them in large doses: three capsules a day to begin with, followed by two later on, are quite sufficient. So you see that even if they were debilitating, which they're not, they couldn't weaken anybody in such small doses.'

My audience relaxes. Now to tackle the question of becoming resistant to antibiotics. I wish I knew who had put this nonsense into people's heads.

'No antibiotic can build up a resistance in the organism which absorbs it. This is a common misapprehension which began with penicillin. Actually, it's the microbes which may develop a resistance or tolerance to antibiotics, but even this is true only of particular microbes and particular antibiotics.

'The antibiotic I propose to give you won't build up any resistance whatever in the germs, and should you need it in future for another reason, you'll find it just as effective as if you'd never taken it.'

'But why didn't you give Miss C. an antibiotic, in that case? She was the one who suggested we came to you.'

My visitors knew all about Miss C.'s treatment ... it's extraordinary how these prescriptions are passed around by word of mouth. 'You gave Mrs X. such-and-such a medicine which completely cured her; but when I tried it, it didn't work.' Of course it didn't – her illness bore no relation to yours! Never try doing that. Medicaments are not cure-alls. Never borrow your friend's ointment; until your illness has been properly diagnosed it's better to do nothing than to experiment in the dark. At best, you won't do yourself any actual harm, but you'll be wasting time which might have been spent having the proper treatment and during which your trouble will be developing unchecked; at worst, the treatment which worked wonders for your friend will be actively detrimental: I've seen cases where an ordinary cold sore has become horribly inflamed after a patient had experimented with a hydrocortisone cream. Preparations belonging to this category should never be applies to a cold sore or herpes.

'Miss C.'s spots', I tell my visitors, 'were quite different from this young man's. You know her and you've seen what they're like, so I'm not giving away any professional secrets. She had small superficial pustules, as they're called, and antibiotics have little effect on spots of this kind. I've occasionally given antibiotics to young girls during the first two months of treatment with the pill, before its beneficial effects have had time to show, in order to calm down spots because they were troubling the patient more than the closed comedones which caused them. But I never prescribe them unless I can be sure, from the kind of spots they are, of being able to calm them down. Antibiotics aren't good for everything and one has to know which ones to use, how to use them, in which cases they'll be effective and what one can expect from them.

'As they don't affect the causes of the disease, seborrhea and closed comedones, but only the consequences, the spots, antibiotics merely interrupt the development of the latter. When you stop using them, the spots come back. That is another reason why they must be taken over long periods.'

Failing a pill for men, one can also, in certain rare cases, have recourse to X-ray treatment.* But this must be given by trained radiologists with experience of this particular form of treatment, which is valid only in those subjects – of both sexes, incidentally – whose acne has ceased to develop in an acute form; in other words, in adult sufferers only, and not even in all of them. X-rays are not a miracle cure any more than antibiotics.

* Not usual practice in Britain. (Tr)

ACNE SURGERY: COMEDONE EXPULSION

In all cases, in men as well as women, the skin must be purged of its closed comedones, and this can be a very tedious process.

As I emphasised earlier on, the closed comedones responsible for acne spots never disappear once they have formed. It's very important to grasp this point: not even the pill will make them disappear in women; it only prevents new ones from forming, and existing ones, once extracted, from reforming. Thus, unless they're removed, patients will have the same stock at the end of their treatment as they had to begin with. Closed comedones have to be eliminated, one by one. But just as the best internal treatment won't lead to a successful result without their removal, it's equally fruitless to extract them without the accompaniment of suitable internal or external remedies.

The correct method of extracting a closed comedone is to open it with a very fine stylet which leaves no mark. *Never squeeze a closed comedone without opening it first; then, once opened, it must be completely evacuated.* Failure to observe these rules results in the remedy being worse than the disease: when one squeezes a closed comedone without opening it, most of its fatty content is forced into the dermis; the result is inflammation of the skin and the formation of deep-seated spots which take weeks to disappear.

That's why *people who squeeze their blackheads or their spots are incurable no matter what one does*, and why, in my opinion, the so-called comedo-extractor is a dangerous instrument. Its place is in the dustbin, not the dressing-table.

The first session of comedone expulsion can take up to half an hour. It requires considerable patience on the part of the operator and endurance on the part of the 'victim'. Nonetheless, it's an essential procedure and I've seldom come across a patient, boy or girl, who will not submit to it bravely once they realise the necessity and understand that the operator is motivated by a desire to help rather than sadism.

As a rule several sessions are required during the course of treatment of acne. Recently, however, the procedure has been greatly facilitated by the discovery of a product derived from vitamin A known as retinoic acid; this substance has the remarkable property of evacuating blackheads and closed comedones. No less than 900 kilograms of it are sold in the U.S.A. every year;

since it's active at a strength of 50 milligrams to 100 grams of cream, this represents the manufacture and consumption of sixty million 30-gram units a year in the U.S.A. – an indication of its success.*

TABLE I   *Summary of treatments inhibiting seborrhea and acne*

Internal treatments	Women	Men
The pill	Yes	No
Antibiotics[1]	Yes	Yes
Vaccines	No	No
Diets	No	No
Vitamins	No	No

External treatments	Women	Men
Acne surgery	Yes	Yes
Peeling[2]	Yes	Yes
Water-in-oil emulsion cream	Yes	No
Cleansing milk	Yes	Sometimes
Retinoic acid	Yes	Yes
Mild soap (super fatted)	No	Yes
Acid detergents	No	No
De-greasing agents[3]	No	No
Sulphur	No	No
Cortisone and its derivatives	No	No
Ultra-violet rays	No	No
X-rays[4]	Sometimes	Sometimes

1   Only in the case of deep-seated spots
2   When treatment is completed
3   Alcohol, ether or acetone base
4   After the age of twenty

* Retinoic acid is now available in the United Kingdom on medical prescription. (Tr)

F

Its only disadvantage is that it can act as an irritant, especially in the early stages of treatment. It must therefore be used with care; with that proviso, however, it makes the extraction of closed comedones considerably less onerous and often unnecessary. True, large deep-seated cysts won't respond to it, but when correctly used it leaves fewer to deal with, while those which remain are easier to extract.

All the remedies I've just outlined are medical treatments in the strict sense of the term: they require a doctor's prescription and should be used only under his supervision. The same applies to peeling, which I haven't overlooked; because of its importance and the fact that its indications aren't limited to acne, I intend to devote a separate chapter to it.

Aside from these treatments, people can do much to help themselves by avoiding useless remedies such as diets or vitamins, or harmful practices such as de-greasing their skin, using preparations containing sulphur, squeezing their blackheads or over-exposing their skin to ultra-violet rays — whether the natural rays of the sun or the artificial rays of a sun-lamp.

If I seem to be repeating myself, it's because experience has taught me that some things cannot be said too often. I've already referred to the sun twice and, at the risk of appearing obsessive, I'm about to refer to it again. The dermatologist is well-placed to judge its so-called beneficial effects, not only in the case of seborrhea but in many other cases which I shall deal with in the next chapter.

3 Degenerative changes in the skin

Although it may last up to an advanced age, seborrhea and its complications are above all a problem of youth, principally affecting adolescents and young adults. Its frequency diminishes after the age of thirty, the age when the various signs of deterioration begin to develop, the victims of which throng the consulting rooms of dermatologists and the cubicles of beauty-parlours — or 'clinics' as they sometimes pompously call themselves.

Male skin, being tougher than female skin, takes longer to show signs of wear and tear. But this time-scale apart, men suffer to the same degree as women, even if they tend to worry about it less. Skin deterioration takes more than one form. These changes differ not only in their visible effects but also in their causes. Some, such as wrinkles, are merely unaesthetic and not skin diseases; others, such as broken veins, not only affect the looks but are also a disease, albeit perfectly benign.

THE EFFECTS OF THE SUN

Of all the skin's many potential enemies, the greatest is the sun. This star, composed entirely of gases, with a luminous layer reaching 6 thousand degrees Centigrade, emits a complex system of rays which take 8 minutes, 18 seconds to travel the 150 million or so kilometres which separate it from the Earth. This system includes several kinds of radiation: luminous rays which give us light; invisible, or infra-red rays which are longer in wave-length and give us heat: rays whose calorific strength, when concentrated on one spot by a magnifying glass, can easily set light to paper or dry wood; and *ultra-violet* rays, which are also invisible but shorter in wave-length than the former.

It is these ultra-violet rays which concern the holiday-maker because, by stimulating the manufacture of pigment in specialised cells called 'melanocytes' (in medical terms, pigment is called 'melanin'), they cause the skin to tan. But they don't concern the holiday-maker alone. They interest the dermatologist too, because of the skin troubles for which they are responsible.

Personally, I'm convinced that if women were to cease exposing themselves to the sun the way they have for the past thirty years since the disastrous fashion for a deep, brown, uniform tan first caught on, dermatologists would lose at least a quarter of their patients and beauty-salons more than half their clients.

I've long proclaimed that the least we dermatologists should do to show our gratitude is to club together and build, as the Aztecs of Mexico did before they were decimated by Cortés and his men, a splendid monument with, on its base, the legend: 'We dermatologists salute you, O Sun!'

It's asking for trouble, these days, to tell a woman she shouldn't sun-bathe. Her reaction is one of hurt and outrage: 'What on earth will people take me for?' she groans, looking tragic.

'If they've got any sense,' I reply, 'they'll take you for someone who wants to keep her skin youthful-looking for as long as possible. Don't misunderstand me, I'm not forbidding you to sun-bathe at all. You can roast your backside until it smokes if you feel so inclined: the worst that can happen is that you won't be able to sit down for a week and you'll have to sleep on your stomach because you'll have blisters and a bottom as red as a baboon's.' Such ravages pass without any long-term consequences. In our climate we only expose our bodies, whether in bathing trunks, bikinis, monokinis or for that matter nothing at all, for thirty days of the year at most as far as the majority of people are concerned, perhaps twice that amount in the case of a privileged few. For the remainder of the year clothes protect our bodies from dangerous rays.

It's a different matter where the face is concerned: exposed to the elements, completely unprotected, from the first day of our lives to the last and handicapped by the resulting increased susceptibility, any additional damage is the last straw. And what goes for the face is also true, to a slightly lesser extent, for the neck, throat and the backs of the hands; but at least we don't always go around bare-chested, and we can wear gloves or put our hands in our pockets. We can't put our noses in our pockets, and this protuberance acts like a magnet to the sun's rays. True, there are such things as nose-shields, but not cheek-shields, or forehead-shields, or chin-shields. And not only do we do nothing to protect our individual masterpiece, our face, from the constant threat of destruction, we actually cover it with stuff to encourage it to turn brown ... including, believe it or not, udder cream!

Until two years ago, I thought I'd seen everything that women's genius could invent for the purpose of destroying their faces.

I've seen faces mottled with dirty grey patches following the application of sun-tan preparations containing oil of bergamot, which is an ingredient in perfume. This pigmentation produces the most striking effect one could wish for, and, moreover, it is 'fast': oil of bergamot, like lavender, is a 'photosensitiser', which means that it makes the skin sensitive to ultra-violet rays, accelerating the formation of pigment and thus giving a faster and deeper tan. The trouble is that this pigmentation is irregular and consequently forms patches which are darker than others. And, to make matters worse, these patches, once formed, never disappear. They pale as the tan fades until they're scarcely noticeable: but the sensitised pigment cells retain the memory of their sensitisation to ultra-violet rays; and every year, at holiday time, they stand out with the same intensity in the same places with the first rays of the sun. A friend of mine has had ample opportunity over the past twenty-two years to appreciate the effects of this brilliant cosmetic idea.

I've also come across some particularly splendid examples of irritated skin in women obsessed with cleanliness which were caused by various additives to the water in which they washed. One patient of mine had been using soda crystals, an example so far unique in my experience. On the other hand, I've got a collection of case-histories of women who had washed their faces in the sort of detergents guaranteed to get your clothes 'whiter than white', as the advertisements say; presumably they thought these products would get their skin 'whiter than white' as well!

I also remember an energetic young woman who, dissatisfied with the state of her complexion, gave her face a good scrubbing with a loofah! What better! And another who ended up as a fine case of eczema as a result of her habit of using sticking plaster on her face every night in order to keep the skin taut, in the hope — unfulfilled, I need hardly add — of preventing wrinkles. While I'm aware that Sacher Masoch has his female disciples and that many women possess masochistic traits, to spend whole nights with sticking plaster tugging at one's skin seems a little extreme!

However it wasn't until I was told about a marvellous sun-tan cream which was all the rage and which was, in fact, udder cream, that I was truly flummoxed. Firstly because I could see no connection whatever between a cow's udder and a woman's face, and secondly because grease – for that was basically all it was – had long been on sale in purified form in chemists' shops, and I could see no reason to use this kind of product on one's skin. Moreover, this absurd procedure of exposing the skin to the sun covered in grease seemed to me to be like nothing so much as cooking the skin in its own juice, and I could see no advantage in that – quite the contrary, in fact.

Once the winter sports season or the summer holiday period is over, I see the results of these deplorable practices in the faces of patients or friends.

One evening I met the young wife of a colleague, just back from skiing; her face was not so much brown as mahogany-coloured; the skin was completely dried up and covered in a network of tiny lines; every feature was accentuated. Normally a very attractive twenty-seven year old, that evening she looked like a wizened old crone.

I don't mind admitting that the sight of a beautiful healthy young woman gives me real pleasure and it exasperates me to see someone who is pointlessly ruining her looks. It's not merely a waste, it's sheer stupidity. I tend to be brutally frank on such occasions. As we left the dining-room I remarked pleasantly: 'Evelyne, have you any idea what a sight you look?' And without giving her a chance to get her breath back for a retort, I led her to a mirror and began to explain what I meant by my blunt remark.

I've often noticed that, where their looks are concerned, people tend to see themselves in terms of clichés until you draw their attention to the facts. For example, wrinkles are supposed to be ageing, so the least little line takes on an importance out of all proportion to reality. A tan, on the other hand, is supposed to make you look healthy; so the browner you are the better and more glamorous you look; we have become blind to what is really happening: that an exaggerated tan makes the features look harder, older and more lined.

If the ageing effect of the sun on the face were confined to the short term, that is for as long as its immediate effects lasted, then relatively little harm would be done.

Unfortunately, ultra-violet rays are a major factor in the actual ageing of the deeper layers of the skin. We now know that they are the principal cause of many degenerative changes previously attributed to age. I'm not suggesting that age doesn't play a part: in the long run, of course, it takes its toll of our skin, as of all our other tissues and organs. The machine gradually wears out with time, but ultra-violet rays considerably accelerate the wear and tear on its surface.

This is especially noticeable in people with open-air jobs who are constantly exposed to the ravages of the sun: no one would call a thirty to thirty-five year old farm-worker, ski-instructor or fisherman an old man, but it's common to find young men in these groups whose facial skin looks twice its age.

Sun-damaged skin may be unavoidable in some professions — it's difficult to imagine a tough trawlerman anointing himself with protective creams — but there's no excuse for white-collar workers, more and more of whom are needlessly suffering the same effects.

The damage to the deeper layers of the skin caused by ultra-violet rays takes years to manifest itself. It comes about in much the same way as that caused by X-rays. We know that an overdose of X-rays can produce irreversible skin changes, conditions known as 'radiodermatitis', which may be delayed for as long as fifteen or even twenty years without producing any visible effects in the meantime.

With the sun's rays, too, years can go by without any apparent reaction; then, suddenly, the skin begins to deteriorate. It happens without warning. One day you can look at yourself in the mirror with equanimity, complacency even; the next, it reflects a very different image: there's a hint of slackness along the jawline, a few wrinkles at the outer corner of the eyelids, the beginnings of a fold in place of the faint line that runs from the nose to the corner of the mouth.

This is the dreaded *coup de vieux*, the insidious onset of a new phase in our lives. If it happens when we're fifty-five, or even fifty, we don't exactly welcome it — few of us are sufficiently philosophical for that — but we can accept it. But if it happens when we're thirty-eight or forty, at the age when the first signs appear in dedicated sun-worshippers, we resent it as being unfair, an unacceptable blow of fate.

This is especially true of our present civilisation when, thanks to the progress of hygiene and preventive medicine, a forty year old woman in good health isn't in the least 'past it'. On the contrary, she's full of vitality and there's not the slightest reason why she should retire from the scene when her continued health and vigour make her perfectly capable of holding her own.

THE EFFECTS OF THE MENOPAUSE

And this is also true of menopausal women. The depressing notion most women have of the menopause is inherited from a past which they still find difficulty in shaking off, just as they're still struggling to emerge from the position of inferiority to which they've been relegated for thousands of years.

These two notions, of the woman who is past-it-at-the-menopause and the woman-as-object, are closely linked. It wasn't so long ago that a woman was considered to be a man's servant and her essential role to provide him with heirs. It's not so surprising, then, that the loss of her principal function, that of reproduction, caused her to lose value in men's eyes and seemed to be the end of everything where she was concerned.

Although now treated as equals, although no longer thought of simply as brood-mares, many women still retire into the background after the menopause as though it represented the beginning of the end, instead of seeing in it the opportunity for a new start in the context of an existence freed from the ties of child-bearing. The 'liberation of women', *pace* certain excitable modern suffragettes, isn't confined to the right to control one's fertility; it also has a lot to do with a fundamental rethinking of ideas concerning the menopause.

These ideas are relatively recent. The problems of the menopause didn't trouble the Romans under Nero or Titus: during the first century of the Christian era the average expectation of life was limited to twenty-three years. And 1200 years later, in the Middle Ages, people knew nothing of the decline in the function of the ovaries because they seldom lived beyond the age of thirty-three. It wasn't until the beginning of the twentieth century, when the average life-span in Western countries had reached forty-eight to fifty years, that a sufficiently large proportion of women were living long enough for the menopause to become a significant problem in our society.

Since then, longevity has been on the increase, and with it the population of women over fifty.

About 25 per cent of menopausal women continue to produce

female hormones in sufficient quantities to spare them the characteristic disorders following the loss of hormones vital to the proper physical, psychological and sexual equilibrium of every woman.

For the remaining 75 per cent — in other words, the great majority of women — the disappearance of the female hormone is almost total; and this creates an abnormal condition which they must endure for the rest of their lives, some twenty-five to thirty years, or, given the expectation of life today, the equivalent of a third or more of their existence.

The onset of this condition is manifested by a profound upheaval in the various systems previously controlled by the female hormone, as a result of which:

1 The skin loses what remains of its elasticity, becoming 'crepy', lax, dried up and scaly; lines become deeply etched;
2 The breasts become slack, the nipples flatten and lose their erectile property;
3 Pubic and under-arm hair becomes fine and sparse; the fatty tissue of the pubis and vulva diminishes;
4 Lastly, the bones become brittle, which explains both the prevalence of hip fractures in elderly women and the shrinkage of the spinal column with a consequent loss of up to twelve centimetres in height.

And these are only those changes which visibly affect the looks. There are many more affecting the muscles, the nervous system, the heart and the arteries.

The dogmatic, negative attitude which persists in treating the menopause as a natural phenomenon fails to take into account these serious degenerative changes, all of which can now easily be prevented by the regular intake of the required amount of female hormone; this treatment, known as hormone replacement therapy, is increasingly popular in America; it allows women who have reached the menopause to keep their faculties, their looks and their vitality intact.

There's no longer any reason for women, like their grandmothers before them, to accept the menopause as a fate to be suffered stoically and in silence; nor need they resign themselves to a faster decline because of it, not even that of their skin — only too sorely tried, as a rule, by repeated and injudicious sun-bathing since adolescence.

The fact is that long before the arrival of the menopause, the majority of women have done everything necessary, summer after summer, to age their skin prematurely, forgetting, in the pleasure of roasting themselves, that *what you do after the age of twenty determines the skin you will have at forty*.

I quite realise how difficult it is for a twenty-year-old to visualise what she will be like at the age of forty: at twenty, forty seems impossibly distant. It's only natural for young people to ignore the future, to seize each passing moment and live it to the full without a thought for the morrow. Between twenty and sixty there's the world of difference in our love of life and, above all, our love of self. The more time passes, the more what remains is precious to us, while the importance we attach to the physical self increases as fast as we deteriorate.

Alas, scarcely are we aware of it than we have reached the day when our age-group acquires an epithet: we have become 'staid' forty-year-olds, 'respected' fifty-year-olds; with any luck, we may even be thought 'well-preserved'. All the more reason why, in order to qualify for these consolation prizes and avoid having the worn face of a sixty-year-old at forty, we should take a few basic precautions.

Types of progressive skin damage that can be attributed to the sun are so numerous they deserve a dermatological treatise to themselves. They range from the purely cosmetic to the badly diseased. In Australia, for instance, the late Professor Belisario of Sydney, a leading specialist in skin cancer, clearly established that the frequency of facial cancers among white populations is greater the sunnier the climate in which they live. That is why there are many more instances of facial skin cancer in Australia than in northern Europe. Moreover, fair-haired people and red-haired people with fair skins are distinctly more vulnerable than dark-haired people whose skins are richer in pigment.

Cancerous degeneration and other equally serious skin diseases do not, of course, come within the scope of this book. Happily, they are relatively rare, especially in our climate, compared to the many medically-speaking benign changes which are the price we have to pay for easily avoidable mistakes. These changes affect us all and they're important not only because they're so common but also because of the psychological repercussions which follow from their unsightliness: I've yet to see the woman who can watch with equanimity as her face or the backs of her hands become mottled with brown marks, and it is interesting to note that more and more men, too, are beginning to worry about them.

The reasons for this kind of skin damage are brought home to us with the realisation that the sun's rays, as well as being essential to life on Earth, are also deadly: ultra-violet rays kill living cells, a property which is actually exploited in the sterilisation of places such as operating theatres.

True, the skin is able to protect itself: its defence is the skin-tan. The pigment manufactured by the melanocytes found among the cells of the basal layer of the epidermis is dispersed throughout the epidermal cells in the form of minute brown or black granules. The greater the amount of pigment manufactured and dispersed, the browner the skin and also the greater the degree of protection: a skin which doesn't tan easily is much less well-protected.

However deep your tan, it won't give you complete protection, as anyone can see for himself from the immediate consequences of sun exposure as well as the delayed skin-changes this provokes. In the course of a summer's intensive sun-bathing, the colour of the skin becomes progressively greyer due to the thickening and drying up of the horny layer of the epidermis.

As we have seen in the preceding chapter, this thickening also affects the sebaceous pores, causing them to become blocked in anyone suffering from seborrhea, encouraging the formation of closed comedones, and thus aggravating acne.

The drying-up of the skin results in the shedding of horny cells known as 'squames' (which is why we talk of the desquamation of the skin); true, the skin doesn't peel off in strips as after sunburn, but in tiny powdery particles; furthermore, when one looks closely, the cutaneous surface appears to be criss-crossed with fine lines, like crackleware china, foreshadowing the crinkled look of old age. This is because it has lost its elasticity: once the keratin in the horny cells has dried up, the skin shrinks and becomes brittle.

Except for acne sufferers, these changes are not very serious in themselves in the short term. During the weeks following exposure to the sun, the desquamation stops and the epidermis appears to recover its former texture and appearance.

However, this apparent recovery is merely superficial and temporary. Gradually, the thickening of the horny layer tends to become a permanent feature; and that means that the equilibrium between the superficial layers of dead cells (remembering that horny cells are dead cells) and the deeper layers of living epidermal cells has been irretrievably upset.

THE AGEING SKIN

This imbalance is accompanied by a thinning of the epidermis as a whole which is one — although far from the most important or visible — of the characteristics of ageing skin.

Further disasters will occur in the epidermis, and also in the dermis, for no layer of the skin is immune.

LENTIGINOSES

The best-known visible sign of an ageing skin is the development of flat, brown maculae, most commonly on the hands, varying in number, size and shape. The old-fashioned, popular word for them was 'liver spots'. They are sometimes known in medical terminology as 'senile' lentiginoses, because of their association with age; but since they can form prematurely in people who work in the open air, they are also closely associated with the activity of ultra-violet rays. For this reason I prefer to call them 'solar' lentiginoses, which is more exact as well as considerably less demoralising. Nevertheless, they are particularly distressing evidence of premature ageing of the skin due to the sun.

KERATOSES

Somewhat less common are 'senile' keratoses, renamed 'solar' keratoses for the same reason. These are brownish-red marks which become rough to the touch. From time to time they shed a dry scale, when another will form to be shed in its turn. Whereas 'solar' lentiginoses are benign, 'solar' keratoses are frankly less so, *for they constitute a pre-cancerous condition.* They are a serious rather than a merely aesthetic problem and I shall discuss them in detail in the next chapter.

But it's in the dermis, the skin's supportive tissue and, as we have seen, its most vital layer, where the nutritive vessels, glands and nerve-endings are located and the exchange of nutrients and gases between blood and cells takes place, that the most irremediable cosmetic damage occurs.

WRINKLES

The connective tissue undergoes changes which affect both the mass of interlocking fibres and the ground substance which coats them, rather as a stiffening coats the fibres of a fabric. The 'mattress' on which the epidermis rests loses its firmness, its resilience. It becomes slack, and it is this slackness which causes wrinkles to form: these are not, as is commonly thought, superficial lines; they are folds made as the epidermis sinks into the depressions in the dermis (as a pillow-case follows the indentations of a rumpled pillow) at places determined by the movements or contractions of muscles beneath the skin. At the same time, the elastic fibres intermingled with the connective fibres in the dermis undergo chemical changes which cause them to lose their elasticity and fragment: consequently the skin loses its suppleness and tone. When pinched, it takes an abnormally long time to regain its shape. It becomes 'perished' like an old piece of elastic ribbon, and lax, with an annoying tendency to obey the laws of gravity and drop: a phenomenon especially noticeable on the eyelids and along the jaw-line, where the cheeks sag to form jowls.

In some areas, the degeneration of the elastic fibres, 'elastosis', is marked by highly characteristic lesions:

1 On the neck, tiny yellowish-white papules form, giving it the appearance of chicken-skin;
2 The temples and cheeks become speckled with minute dry black spots and tiny pimples which look like the blackheads and closed comedones formed in acne but are nothing of the kind.

Every dermatologist has seen thousands of skin conditions like these, and not only in elderly people. They are dressed up, in current jargon, by epithets as varied as they are freakish: we have 'demoisturised' skin, skin which 'can't breathe', 'devitalised' skin. All such notions are totally meaningless.

A skin cannot become demoisturised! This often surprises people; their heads have been crammed with moisturising creams, moisturing lotions, to the point where they actually believe that they can have demoisturised skin.

I shall come back to this important point later, with reference to so-called 'dry' skin—which doesn't exist either, dermatologically speaking, but which does have certain points in common with the epidermal surface of ageing skin.

And to say that a skin is devitalised is a contradiction in terms: to be devitalised means to be made lifeless, i.e. dead. However advanced its age, a skin is not dead while the organism to which it belongs is alive. It dies only when the organism dies. By the same token I would dearly like to know what manufacturers mean when they claim that their products have the remarkable property of 'revitalising' the skin.

As for the skin which 'can't breathe', I've no idea what this means or what it's supposed to be: respiration, to the best of my knowledge, is a function of the lungs. To say that a skin cannot breathe is therefore patent nonsense.

True, exchanges do take place through the skin between the interior and exterior environments: water is eliminated invisibly* through the epidermal barrier and evaporates in the surrounding air, combining with the visible sweat to cool the cutaneous surface and control the internal temperature.

The skin also eliminates carbon dioxide gas which helps to maintain its surface acidity and its resistance to the action of alkaline substances (such as soda).

As I've already pointed out, in the context of the functions of the skin, if such exchanges are prevented from taking place because large areas of the skin have been coated with some impermeable substance, the whole body may suffer as a result. But this has nothing whatsoever to do with the skin itself being unable to breathe.

ATROPHIC SKIN

The adjective which comes nearest to describing ageing skin is atrophic, which means a diminution in volume, without defining the *cause* of the diminution: a skin may be atrophic because it has suffered senile involution; it can also be atrophic where there is a scar left by a severe burn.

Beyond a certain point, you cannot reverse an ageing, atrophic skin. You don't call the fire-brigade after the fire has consumed everything, you call them at the first sign of flames; or, better still you take sensible precautions to prevent fire from breaking out in the first place.

* This phenomenon is known as 'insensible perspiration'. (A-B)

Of course, you cannot avoid the unavoidable: the skin will age eventually, sun or no sun, and on the face a little sooner than elsewhere; what matters is that it shouldn't age before its time and that it should age as slowly, as late and as little as possible. And this isn't wishful thinking; I still occasionally meet women born at the end of the last century who followed the fashion of their youth for white skin, greatly aided by sunbonnets and parasols, and who have been spared the worst effects of ageing such as I've just described; in spite of their years they still have hardly any wrinkles and are blessed with clear, fresh complexions which are a pleasure to see.

That's why I take every opportunity to preach to young women the wisdom of shading the face with a sunshade, wearing a wide-brimmed hat and using sun-screen creams; and I forbid them to use sun-tan preparations.

I also remind them that a sun-screen cream or lotion can never give you complete protection, regardless of what the label might say. All they have to do is to be patient, and some ultra-violet rays will get through: always too many, in my opinion, but certainly enough to reassure those who are terrified they may return from holiday the colour of an aspirin tablet.

Nor do sun-screen preparations give long-term protection: what you put on at ten in the morning will be useless by midday, the most dangerous time of all. You must re-apply it every hour and a half to two hours, depending on the heat, the wind and how much you perspire, all of which help to dry it up or wash it off; and, needless to say, every time you have swum in the sea or a pool. This means having it constantly with you, in your beach-bag, in the pocket of your anorak, and remembering to use it. I grant you that this requires a certain amount of self-discipline, but it's worth it.

And I'm glad to say that more and more women seem prepared to accept these petty restrictions with good grace; they may be a little sad, at the end of their summer or skiing holiday, not to have the same triumphant, tanned face as their friends, but I can assure them that the day will come when it will be their turn to triumph, thanks to having kept their smooth, fresh complexions, just at the moment when their friends are losing theirs.

In any case, they can always improve on their natural tan by using one of the artificial tanning preparations* which cause the

* The active chemical is Dihydroxacetone. (Tr)

keratin in the epidermis to turn brown through a chemical reaction. Their effect is quite different from that of make-up, since it's the actual substance of the superficial cells of the skin which changes colour, and this won't fade until the cells themselves are eliminated. An artificial tan won't wash off, will last for two or three days depending on the speed of the desquamation of the skin, and is easy to maintain. But since it's a dye and not a pigmentation, it affords no protection whatever against sunburn; it merely offers an easy way of avoiding the contrast between a pale face and a well-tanned body.

I can assure any woman here and now that if she sticks to these rules, she will never, at any stage of her life, look her age.

For those for whom realisation comes too late and who are already showing the tell-tale signs of a fading skin, there are various ways of limiting the damage.

The effectiveness of these methods, and hence their choice, depends on the nature of the damage you are trying to remedy. Broadly speaking this damage can be divided into three stages:

1 The skin is dried up;
2 The skin is dried up, the complexion blotchy due to the onset of thickening of the horny layer, and the dermis has begun to lose its firmness;
3 The skin shows signs of losing its elasticity, with incipient jowls, 'crow's feet', frown and laughter lines and baggy eyelids.

THE TREATMENT OF AGEING SKIN ACCORDING TO THE DEGREE OF SEVERITY

FIRST STAGE: THE SKIN IS DRIED UP

The reader may have noticed that I invariably talk of dried-up skin, rather than dry skin.

There is an excellent reason for this: from the dermatological point of view, dry skin is a myth—it doesn't exist. To understand why this is, a few words on the hydration of cutaneous tissue are necessary.

When describing the skin, I emphasised the fact that all living cells are bathed in a fluid emanating from the blood and lymph and without which they cannot live: this is called 'interstitial' fluid because it circulates in the microscopic spaces or interstices which separate one cell from another. The same is naturally true for all skin cells, with the exception of the superficial, or horny, cells which have lost their nucleus and are dead.

If the layer of horny cells is torn and the uppermost layers of living cells exposed, a slight seepage of this interstitial fluid occurs — as everyone knows who has suffered a graze or minor burn. This oozing seldom lasts long because the fluid coagulates and forms a scab, beneath which the scar will eventually be sited.

No drop of water from the exterior ever reaches the skin's living cells; between them and the horny cells on the surface there is an impervious barrier; and this is just as well, otherwise the consequences would be disastrous. On the other hand, since water is constantly passing from the interior to the exterior, the horny cells, although situated outside what I have called the 'interior lake', are, in normal conditions, continually impregnated with water: the 'insensible perspiration' which is imperceptible, and the visible sweat which flows over their surface.

This process is all-important, because the correct balance of the horny cells depends on their hydration: the water gives them their suppleness; and when you have a supple horny layer, you have a soft, velvety skin. But there mustn't be too much or too little:

— If in contact with an excess of water over too long a period the horny cells swell until they burst;

— If deprived of water, they shrink and become dried up and brittle. And the more they were formerly impregnated, the more they will shrink; there comes a point where a horny cell which has dried up after having been over-hydrated is damaged beyond repair: the next time there's a flow of water, it will refuse to swell at all.

Horny cells are at one and the same time greedy for water and incapable of retaining it.

The water they have captured from the sweat and invisible perspiration doesn't remain in them indefinitely: it evaporates into the outside air. Catchment and evaporation take place continuously: the correct balance of a horny cell, in terms of its hydration, depends on the balance between these two processes; as long as no more water evaporates than is trapped, this balance is assured. But it can be upset in a number of different ways.

The two principal causes of the horny cells drying up are the de-greasing of the skin and the dryness of the surrounding air.

G

Here we come to a cardinal point: contrary to general belief, fats, whether natural or not, are incapable by themselves of restoring suppleness to horny cells which have dried up. *They act preventively by inhibiting, through their impermeability, the evaporation of water trapped in the horny cells.* The fats in the sebum act in the same way. If the secretion of the sebaceous glands which produce these fats is insufficient, or if it's destroyed by injudicious practices, such as soaping the face or using alcohol-based lotions, then nothing will prevent evaporation from continuing unchecked; the degree of humidity in the air plays an important part in this process; the lower it is, the greater the tendency of the water to escape from the horny cells. That is why they dry up more in winter, especially in buildings without proper humidification to compensate for the effects of central heating.

As I've just pointed out, when these cells dry up, they shrink. Consequently, the entire horny layer will also shrink, diminish in volume and contract over the layers of living cells immediately beneath it; now, these cells never alter in volume, because of the interstitial fluid that ensures their permanent, invariable hydration. The result is that they are compressed into the shrunken horny layer which encloses them. This process is felt as a tugging sensation, and can even produce a burning sensation if the horny layer, brittle through being dried up, should crack under the pressure as the living epidermal cells strive to free themselves from the vice which grips them.

Not only this, but once the dehydrated horny cells burst the cutaneous surface becomes a constellation of minute prickles, invisible to the naked eye but rough to the touch.

To sum up, so-called dry skin is in reality 'rough' skin whose basic characteristic is the disjunction of the horny layer and its cells.

All types of skin can become rough and dried up, even oily skin if de-greased too harshly and too often. But normal skin is clearly the most vulnerable of all because, unless one is careful, its balance can so easily be tipped towards a dried-up condition by sun, cold and wind.

The management of dried-up skin

Whether it's a question of preventing skin from becoming dried up or correcting it afterwards, the methods are the same.

These methods are straightforward and flow logically from the situation I've just described. The principle underlying them can be summed up as follows: *it is more effective to prevent the horny layer from becoming dehydrated than it is to hydrate it.*

Of course, one can re-hydrate the horny cells by wetting them. But the effect of such artificial hydration is negligible when compared with that of insensible perspiration: in a temperate climate this amounts to four to six hundred grams of water, or an average of half a litre a day, traversing the horny layer of the skin, quite apart from the visible sweat which flows over its surface. And in a tropical climate these figures can reach eight to ten litres a day!

To achieve the same results by artificial means, you would have to wet the skin continuously: invisible and visible perspiration are continuous processes which ensure the permanent hydration of the horny cells. Clearly, a wetting for two or three minutes night and morning is not going to replace natural hydration. Not only can it not replace it, but if care is not taken to avoid over-saturating the horny cells it can be dangerous: if they become over-saturated they will burst, and, *if the water is not prevented from evaporating immediately afterwards*, the horny layer will become abruptly dried-up.

I wonder who first thought it was a good idea to spray water on to the face and leave the damp skin to dry in the air. This practice is guaranteed to produce an unpleasant tugging sensation for the reasons I have just described and, ultimately, to accelerate the degeneration of the skin.

The one thing you must never do is to leave your skin to dry: whenever you wet it, you should dry it carefully to keep saturation within limits, and then put on a cream to prevent evaporation.

But what kind of cream?

'Moisturising' creams

The older I get, the more wary I become of these elegant, light creams which are, it must be admitted, pleasant to use. They are the same oil-in-water emulsions I mentioned earlier in the context of oily skin.

Despite their richness in water, their moisturising effect is nil because the water evaporates very rapidly. Moreover, their fat content is insufficient to give the skin any valid protection against the drying-up of the horny cells. Consequently, in people with normal skin, they can actually encourage the development of a chronic, extremely uncomfortable dried-up condition.

This is a long-delayed effect, usually observed in women between the ages of thirty and thirty-two who have been using this type of preparation for twelve years or more. As you might expect, the normal skin of a young healthy adult is fairly resistant. But the pitcher can go once too often to the well ... and in the end, due to the combination of repeated hygienic and cosmetic errors, this resistance crumbles: the skin gives up the ghost.

People's first reaction is to blame the brand of cream they always use; so they change it, again and again, always without success. Being of the same type, all these preparations share the same defect, which is not one of quality but of unsuitability for the skin to which they're applied.

'But they're good products,' I can hear people object. I wonder why; what justification do they have for saying so?

The answers I get are usually painfully inadequate.

'Because they're well made.'

'I agree, but that goes without saying, I should hope.'

'Because the ingredients are of top quality.'

'Quite true: modern cosmetics are made from first-class ingredients; it would hardly be in the manufacturer's interest to put poor quality goods on the market.'

'Because they don't cause allergies.'

'Any cosmetic sold in huge quantities must obviously be harmless to the majority of women using it, otherwise it wouldn't last long.'

'Because they're pleasant to use.'

'You shouldn't go by appearances, they can be misleading.'

The fact is that none of this goes to the root of the problem: in cosmetics, as in dermatology, a good product is one whose composition is suited to its purpose.

How can one possibly claim that preparations designed for daily use over long periods are equally suitable for oily skin, normal skin, dried-up skin, atrophic skin, when no one has the faintest idea what they contain?

This question is greeted with dead silence. Everyone is stumped! For reasons of commercial security, the formula of a cosmetic preparation is a jealously guarded secret. Even those whose job it is to sell cosmetics only know what the manufacturers, who are free to say anything they please, choose to tell them.

The industry takes full advantage of this state of affairs, and, to justify their attitude, incomprehensible to doctors who fail to see how products whose properties have not been scientifically tested can be recommended, manufacturers claim that their preparations are chemically neutral.

This is a surprising statement, to say the least; if such were really the case, why the variety of products? One should be able to do the work of all. This is obviously not so, and beauty creams are not in the least neutral. Depending on their formula, for instance, they may or may not aggravate seborrhea, may or may not encourage the skin to dry up.

What we need to know, therefore, is how to choose between them.

Unfortunately, as things stand at the moment, there is no valid basis for choice and so women use cosmetics blindly and indiscriminately. No wonder mistakes are made.

As far as 'moisturising' creams are concerned, some women's skin is tougher than others and seems to be able to adapt itself to this particular type of cosmetic without apparent ill-effect. Lucky though such women are, there's nothing to say that they wouldn't be even better off if they left well alone.

'Protective' creams

However that may be, for the majority of women the best method of preventing or treating dried-up skin is to use creams which are emulsions of water-in-oil.

These creams, which contain more fat that water, cover the epidermis with an impermeable film which prevents the water trapped in the horny tissue from evaporating. For dermatological purposes they are defined as covering, emollient, protective and balancing: they are suitable for people with oily skin because, as we have seen in the preceding chapter, they don't provoke reactive seborrhea; they are also suitable for people with normal skin because they don't upset its balance, and for people with dried-up skin because they help to cure this condition.

They are the true 'maids of all work' of cosmetics.

Unfortunately, as far as I've been able to discover, there are not many available on the market.*

The preference shown by cosmetic manufacturers for so-called moisturising creams probably reflects commercial considerations: oil being more expensive than water, the less you use, the lower the manufacturing costs, and the higher the profit margin. A member of a consumers' association even said as much on a French television programme.

It may also reflect marketing considerations: protective creams are slightly less agreeable to use than 'moisturising' creams, and consequently less easy to sell.

At any rate, it certainly doesn't reflect the needs of the consumer, since most women haven't the least idea what these are. What they want is to acquire a good skin and keep it in the best possible condition; and as far as I can see they are ready to do anything in the attempt, no matter how stupid. The same women who, in other circumstances, will exercise their judgment, their critical faculties, lose all common sense when it comes to beauty-care. One patient of mine in particular was a perfect example of this strange failing: she was about fifty years old and owned her own business; ten minutes' conversation was enough for me to realise that here was an exceptionally intelligent, responsible woman; when I expressed my astonishment at her credulity where cosmetics were concerned, a credulity which hardly seemed in character, she replied: 'Yes, I'm perfectly well aware what a fool I am, but I've only got to read about all the marvels they claim to perform and I can't resist buying them; sooner or later I see that the stuff doesn't work, my skin's as bad as ever, and I discover that I've been had yet again.'

The truth is that most women, once they're persuaded that it will do them good, are as happy to use one product as another; personally, I've never known a patient jib at using a protective cream in place of her 'moisturising' cream.

Moreover, the comparison of the results between one and the other is quickly made; even if the 'moisturising' cream in question belongs to that new generation of cosmetics seasoned with fruit or vegetable extracts — as varied as they are useless and ineffective

* In the United Kingdom these products are usually labelled 'all-purpose' or 'cold' creams in the case of the face, and 'barrier' creams in the case of the hands. (Tr)

— which nowadays, for the sake of their imaginary virtues, clutter up the dressing-tables of our wives and girl-friends.

When all's said and done it doesn't really matter if their array of beauty aids looks like a botanical garden as long as the basis of these preparations at least has a structure and a composition which corresponds to the needs of their skin.

Provided that they're harmless, the fact that additives, whether animal or vegetable, possess none of the properties claimed for them in the advertisements is of no concern to the dermatologist; it is rather a matter for legislation.

What does concern him, though, is that the basic ingredients should be suited to their purpose. And it is to be hoped that cosmetic manufacturers, who are past masters at the art of making emulsions of the oil-in-water variety, will bring the same virtuosity and talent to bear on the creation of water-in-oil emulsions which, in the majority of cases, are much to be preferred.

SECOND STAGE: THE SKIN IS DRIED UP, THE COMPLEXION BLOTCHY AND THE RESILIENCE OF THE DERMIS IS AFFECTED

By this stage, ordinary cosmetics are no longer enough and one must have recourse to dermatological treatments. These consist basically of hormone creams and skin-peeling.

Hormone creams

In so far as they are water-in-oil emulsions these creams belong to the same family of cosmetics as the one I've just mentioned in connection with the first stage. But the addition of hormones, in the appropriate amounts, gives them more extensive properties.

It was a leading American endocrinologist (for those who don't know, endocrinology is the speciality dealing with hormonal problems) who proved that the application of sex hormones, whether male or female, stimulates the connective and elastic tissues of the dermis.

As I have laid so much emphasis on the cutaneous barrier which isolates the interior environment from the exterior, it might seem surprising that I am now proposing to introduce foreign substances through the skin. In fact, I'm not contradicting myself: any substance that is soluble in the fats on the cutaneous surface can penetrate the barrier and reach the organism, always providing that its particles are small enough to be able to pass through the microscopic interstices which separate each cell from the next. If the particles are too large they remain on the outside: this is the case with the embryo and placenta extracts which certain cosmetic products are proudly advertised to contain. These extracts, while having undoubted stimulating effects on the cells when given by intramuscular injection, have no such effect when applied to the skin.

Some twenty years ago, I badly disappointed a close woman friend who manufactured 'revitalising' ampoules containing an extract of chicken-embryo for which she claimed rejuvenating properties. In perfectly good faith, I should add: she was profoundly convinced of the truth of her claim and it's a well-known fact that people see what they want to see. Everyone who has been to India has 'seen' a fakir making a rope uncoil upwards from the ground, stiff as a post; but no photograph has yet recorded it — unlike its operator, the camera cannot be influenced. My friend who made the miraculous embryonic extract swore to me that her product worked. I swore the opposite. To settle the matter once and for all, I suggested to her that we set up a scientifically controlled experiment. I found six volunteers, all of whom were between fifty and sixty years old and thus showed signs of the onset of dermal atrophy. At the start of the experiment, before applying the product, I took a small piece of skin from each volunteer for the purposes of comparison; at the end of the experiment I took another small piece, not only from the middle of the treated area but from the identical spot on the opposite, untreated side of the body, in order to exclude any spontaneous change in the skin during the course of the experiment. After two months of applications morning and night, using three times the amount specified, a detailed microscopic examination of the skin samples by a specialist revealed not the smallest difference between the treated and untreated pieces of skin: the microscope proved to be no more suggestible than the camera.

Sex hormones, on the other hand, are able to penetrate the skin with ease: so much so that they are at least as effective when rubbed into the skin as when injected into the muscle in the same quantities.

For this reason, care must be taken not to apply too much when using a hormone cream: the dermis contains special receptors which take up a limited quantity only. As long as this amount is not exceeded, all the hormones remain in the skin and there's no risk of systemic effects, even in the case of prolonged use. This is important, because these creams need to be applied regularly, morning and night, over a period of years, not only to the face, but also to the neck, which deteriorates to the same degree.

Problems at the second stage of ageing don't disappear overnight like a headache after aspirin. They develop slowly and surely with time and the rigours to which the skin is exposed, day after day, year after year. If the treatment is interrupted, the troubles reappear. They must therefore be treated in continuous fashion, always bearing in mind that the treatment works on a day-to-day basis. Given these conditions, one may expect to see visible improvements: by this I mean that the woman who sticks punctiliously to the rules will find that her skin becomes noticeably firmer and more supple, and that her friends, suitably jealous, will tell her how well she looks and ask her how on earth she manages it.

At present, hormone creams cannot be bought ready-made over the counter: they require a doctor's prescription. Legally speaking, a cream containing hormones is a drug, and the marketing of drugs is strictly controlled and requires a pharmaceutical licence.

Since the famous Thalidomide affair* there has been much stricter surveillance by the competent authorities, and, in France, licences are granted only after a commission has studied an expert appraisal which must incorporate scientific verification of the composition of any product containing a drug together with a report of its exact properties, its purpose, its lack of toxicity, its precise description and its method of use. Once legally sanctioned, it may be sold only by chemists and remains liable to periodic inspection by the authorities.

Provisions like these, guaranteeing the safety of the consumer, do not apply to cosmetic or hygienic products, which have never been subjected to any constraint or limitation whatsoever, with the exception of a list of substances, including female hormones, which they are not permitted to contain.

These substances apart, manufacturers may use any ingredient

---

* During the 1960s the Thalidomide drug was responsible for a virtual epidemic of babies deformed at birth; this horrifying potentiality was missed during clinical trials. (A-B)

they choose without being required to furnish either explanation or justification to any authority whatever.

I have always believed that cosmetic manufacturers should be subject to measures which would allow for spot-checks to be made in order to ensure that their products conformed to the claims made for them, both as to their properties and their composition.

If their properties had to be proved, I wouldn't be at all surprised if a number of 'lines' were withdrawn; however, those that passed with flying colours would emerge in a stronger position than ever before.

If the contents were subject to supervision, moreover, then accidents such as that recently where talcum powder caused the death of several infants in a number of countries would be avoided. The substance responsible, hexachlorophane, is an excellent antiseptic and normally completely harmless. In this case, a batch of talcum powder became toxic because it contained twenty times the normal amount of hexachlorophane due to a manufacturing error, and was distributed before anyone was aware of this fact: something that should never have been allowed to happen.

Such accidents are impossible in the pharmaceutical industry, where each batch is numbered and thoroughly tested before leaving the factory. A patient using a drug under his doctor's supervision is completely safe from any untoward tragedy arising out of similar errors.

Not surprisingly, following the general outcry surrounding this deplorable incident, many laboratories were forced to withdraw hexachlorophane products from circulation. Personally, I thought this was going too far: one doesn't shut down the entire railway system because of a single rail disaster. It isn't the hexachlorophane that we should blame; nor is it even the manufacturing error: when machines are controlled by men, human error is always possible.

No, the root of the problem lies at the end of the production line, in the lack of proper surveillance; a campaign should be launched for hygiene products to be brought under the control of the authorities, as in the United States. Then, with as much publicity as had been given to the tragedy, it could be announced that rigorous measures were to be enforced, rendering manufacturers liable under the law, in order to make such accidents impossible in future.

But where hygienic and cosmetic products are concerned there appears to be an 'understanding' — and, naturally, no one would dream of suggesting that this might have something to do with the massive advertising budgets devoted to these products. And this means that the information offered to the public is not always characterised by scientific accuracy or clarity.

I hope I will be forgiven for this digression: I felt there was no harm in getting certain facts into perspective and restating a few truths.

Skin-peeling

Nor are clarity and accuracy exactly the dominant qualities when it comes to the information beauticians whisper in the ear of their clients on the subject of peeling.

Examples of the kind of thing often repeated to me are: 'Peeling consists in removing a skin', 'peeling is dangerous', 'peeling is painful', 'peeling damages the skin'; and, citing someone at second-hand who is supposed to have suffered skin-damage as a result of peeling: 'peeling doesn't work', and 'peeling weakens the skin'. Such inaccuracies only go to prove that the people who bandy them about don't know what they are talking about.

Peeling is not dangerous, or damaging, or painful, or ineffective, or weakening. But neither is it a panacea, a miracle method capable of reversing all types of skin damage, nor a rejuvenating cure for all types of ageing skin.

Like all treatments, it has its limitations. Nevertheless, when there are good and sufficient reasons for doing it, when it is performed by a properly trained practitioner who knows what he's doing, one can confidently say that it is one of the most reliable of dermatological treatments. Depending on the individual, its results will be good, very good or excellent. They will never be non-existent or poor.

But one should not — and I repeat, not — expect more of peeling than it can give, and, in order to know what one is entitled to expect, one must first know what it entails and how it works.

What is peeling?

Inaccuracies abound here, too; peeling means what it says: the process of peeling the skin.

However, there are different methods of making the skin peel:

you can get it to peel if you rub it with a cotton-wool pad soaked in liquid nitrogen or with a stick of carbon dioxide 'snow'. Liquid nitrogen and solid carbon dioxide give off intense cold. Contact with them causes burns accompanied by inflammation, oozing and the formation of scabs, and destroys the epidermal cells—to a greater or lesser depth depending on the strength of the application —by coagulating them with cold in the same way as white of egg is coagulated with heat.

You can also make the skin peel by applying acids to it, such as salicylic acid and trichloracetic acid, which will also destroy the epidermal cells; both the horny cells and, if the acid concentration is high, even the sub-horny cells.

Lastly, you can make the skin peel by exposing it to ultra-violet rays: as we all know, skin peels after sunburn, and the same effect can be obtained with a sun-lamp.

Unna's paste

Skin-peeling, as it is understood by dermatologists, or, for that matter, by its inventor, the German dermatologist Unna who perfected it in 1882, does not involve any of the above procedures.

I mention the date deliberately, in order to remind anyone who needs reminding that not all the best techniques have been developed in the last twenty years.

Nearly a century later not a word needs to be added or altered in Unna's description of his method of peeling, the cases where it should be applied and the effects it produces. He gave it the name of 'exfoliation', a word which should be retained for it describes better than any other what takes place and also helps to distinguish this method of peeling from others which have nothing to do with it.

To exfoliate means literally to take away a leaf, or, in the case of the skin, the fine pellicle which constitutes the horny layer.

The special characteristic of exfoliation technique is that no destruction of the cells is involved. The cells in the horny layer detached from the skin remain absolutely intact. Only a few substances have this property of detaching the horny layer without destroying it, of which one is phenol and a derivative of phenol known as resorcin. Thus, Unna's method is called 'resorcin exfoliation'. It is carried out by means of a paste perfected by its inventor (a paste is a combination of powder and grease); its formula is such that the preparation neither clings to the skin, like Vaseline, nor penetrates it, like lanolin (which is the fat obtained from sheep's wool); it contains 50 grams of resorcin for every 100 grams of a composition based on lard (which is pork fat).

The formula should never be modified: a patient came to see me one day after a terrible experience with peeling: for three days she had had an appalling burning sensation following which thick scabs formed, and it was more than two weeks before the effects subsided. Knowing that Unna's paste never caused violent reactions of the kind, I made enquiries and discovered that in her case a penetrating emulsion had been incorporated into the formula, something which is both contrary to common sense and to the principle of the technique itself.

The technique of exfoliation

This is very simple:

The paste is spread on to the area of the skin to be treated with a spatula and left on for a short period determined by the condition of the skin and the nature of the disorder; how long it takes to apply depends on the operator's skill.

On the face, for instance, it is left on for between fifteen and twenty-five minutes; on the back, one can safely leave it on for thirty to thirty-five minutes.

People undergo this treatment as out-patients: there is no need whatever for hospitalisation, merely a visit to the clinic on two successive days: in my opinion, there should be two successive applications at twenty-four hours' interval.

Not every zone of the skin reacts to the same degree to applications of the same duration: the area around the mouth, for example, is more sensitive than the rest of the face, the forehead in particular; the nape of the neck and the kidney region are more sensitive than the shoulder-blades. It is therefore a good idea on the second day to 'touch up' with paste those points which have reacted less than the others.

When the time has expired the paste is scraped, not washed, off. After this is done the patient will have a burning sensation comparable to that of sunburn. All patients say that this is quite bearable and only lasts two or three hours. A couple of ordinary pain-killers are enough to make it hardly noticeable.

When the patient stands up (having been lying down throughout the treatment), there is often some giddiness, rather like the effect of alcohol on an empty stomach. This is due to the acute congestion of the treated skin and is nothing to be alarmed about: it passes off within a minute or two. To avoid appearing drunk, it's a good idea not to get up too quickly after treatment.

Immediately after an application of resorcin paste the skin is red, or rather purplish, with a slight frosty glint and some puffiness. It is far from being a spectacle to excite undue notice or alarm: you can safely go home on the underground or bus without causing a disturbance. And, for the first two days at least, even your most tactless friends – the sort of people who say 'Good God, what's happened to you?' or 'What in the world have you been doing to yourself!' – will find little to exclaim about. Of course something can be seen, but nothing very dreadful.

After the third day, however, it's another story: the skin takes on a brownish tinge which darkens rapidly to reach its maximum intensity on the fourth day. By this time the face looks like that of a skier who has carelessly omitted to protect himself from the sun and ended up with the degree of sunburn unique to high altitudes.

The difference is, of course, that while sunburn destroys the skin, exfoliation restores it.

At the end of the fourth day desquamation begins on the more mobile areas of the face, usually around the mouth, in the form of large dry strips beneath which the skin appears pink as a baby's.

It continues for the next three days, the nose and outer edges of the face being the last areas to peel. During these final three days, the patient's appearance, half-brown, half-pink, is somewhat clown-like – not, one would think, the ideal moment to choose to go on a round of parties. Yet, about twenty years ago in Paris, I did several successive peelings on a young woman who held an important post in NATO; she had to go to a lot of functions, parties and banquets in the course of her job, and she continued to attend them as though nothing was the matter!

If *daytime* functions are prohibited for the duration of facial exfoliation – for reasons which have nothing to do with the looks, as I shall explain later – evening ones are not.

So my patient went from one official gathering to another coolly indifferent to her temporary appearance and without anyone so much as remarking on it. In fact, I don't believe they really noticed! It's our own attitude towards our disfigurement, whatever it may be, which attracts other people's attention. If we can manage to forget it and behave as though it didn't exist, then no one will pay any attention to it, unless, of course, it happens to be unduly repellent.

There is nothing unpleasant, embarrassing or painful about the process of exfoliation, other than the mild burning sensation following each application.

Nor are there any nasty surprises in store: the pattern is always the same. I have known fine skins to peel completely within five days, but rarely; or, equally rarely, to take as much as eight days; as a general rule, it's all over by the seventh day and you can return to circulation with a fresh complexion and a clear skin.

Sometimes, because of downy skin, especially around the ears, or because of a man's beard, the fine horny squames are impaled and trapped by the hairs. These squames are loose but refuse to fall off, and must thus be removed individually, but with care: one should never remove them prematurely. Any attempt to do so will defeat the object of the treatment and result in damage to the epidermis in the form of hideous red marks which take months to disappear.

Precautions

Those masochists who spend blissful moments night and morning examining themselves in the mirror, preferably a magnifying mirror, for imaginary blackheads while making exaggerated grimaces—now the tongue pushes out the cheek, now the lower lip—the better to 'get at the pores' for pressing, pinching, squeezing and digging, should be warned here and now that such practices, if indulged in during peeling, will lead to catastrophe.

Aside from this risk—which isn't one at all since it depends not on the treatment but the patient's own actions, and is so rare that I've only known one case of a patient who persisted in taking it—there are only two dangers associated with peeling.

Both are connected with the fact that phenol and its derivatives—hence resorcin—are allergy-producing substances which may provoke either contact allergies or photosensitisation.

Phenol eczema

Fortunately, phenols are weak allergens. But weak or not, when they produce an allergic reaction the resulting eczema is just as acute with all the unpleasantness that entails: red, swollen, oozing face and itching that last a week or more; and to make matters worse, the peeling is a failure; one doesn't even have the consolation of a successful outcome.

Prior to peeling, therefore, I consider it a professional duty to do a patch test. This is a simple procedure whereby a small amount of paste is applied behind the ear and left on for ten minutes, as in peeling itself. If there is no reaction within four days, the test can be said to be negative and one can safely proceed. If the test is positive there will be itching and inflammation, reproducing over a tiny area what would have occurred over the treated surface as a whole had one not taken this precaution; as it is limited to a square centimetre of skin hidden behind the ear, the damage is minimal and purely temporary. But all idea of peeling must be given up.

However there's no cause to be discouraged; I've come across only three positive tests in twenty-five years. The chances of triggering a phenol eczema are therefore statistically negligible. But since for someone at risk they amount to a certainty, and, thanks to the test, the risk is easily avoidable, it can never be justified.

Phenol photosensitisation

'Photosensitisation' is simply a special form of allergic reaction, requiring the combined action of the sun and a chemical substance. Alone, neither has any effect, but together they can trigger various reactions. These may take the form of eczema but, more often, they appear as brown marks, in streaks or irregular blots, similar to those which will appear, as I warned earlier, when exposure to the sun has been preceded by an application of scent, eau de cologne or a sun-tan preparation containing oil of bergamot.

Phenols can cause the same ugly pigmentation. After peeling, the pigment becomes concentrated around the edges of the treated areas, especially under the eyes. As with all abnormal pigmentation, it is 'fast' and takes a very long time to fade.

I see no point in undergoing peeling only to end up looking like a chimney-sweep. For this reason patients must not go out of doors in the daytime while peeling is taking place, even if the sky is overcast. Of course it's rather claustrophobic to be shut up indoors for a week when one is perfectly fit, particularly for people who are unable to work at home.

The risk of photosensitisation is not confined to the period of exfoliation; it lasts at least two months. This entails two further precautions: first and foremost, the regular application of a sun-screen preparation throughout this period, regardless of the weather, regardless of the smog polluting the atmosphere over big cities and filtering the ultra-violet rays; the skin must have constant protection – even on journeys to and from the office or the shops. Second, *the strict avoidance of sunny climates*; this is why peeling should never be undertaken in summer and why, in winter, holidays in the mountains should be avoided. I don't know of a single case where these warnings have been ignored with impunity; the result is always and inevitably the necessity for further prolonged treatment to get rid of the pigmentation, not to mention total abstention from sun-bathing for a long time.

Women's irresponsibility in such matters is amazing! Before the militant feminists jump down my throat, I'll explain why I say women and not men: in this particular instance, men are far less reckless than women, possibly because they're more pusillanimous; men either follow instructions to the letter, or else ignore peeling altogether. Women either interpret the rules as they see fit, or forget some or all of them, or remember them, but too late!

I discharged one such woman patient last year; she was thoroughly briefed and delighted with the results of her peeling; continuing care appeared to present no problem since it was March and she wasn't due to go on holiday until August: 'You needn't worry, doctor, there's no danger; it's five months before I go to the Côte d'Azur ... ' At the end of May I received an anguished telephone call; she had to see me at once. My secretary arranged an emergency appointment and I found myself confronted with a face mottled with the irregular dirty-grey patches typical of photosensitisation.

'You've been in the sun, in spite of everything I told you,' I accused her.

'No, doctor, I promise you I've been very careful.'

At this, I exploded. Nothing makes me angrier than to see a successful treatment ruined through carelessness. Moreover, it was obvious that she was prevaricating.

'That's not true; you couldn't have developed pigmentation like that unless you'd been exposed to the sun. There really isn't any point in doing a peeling only to have this happen. It's sheer vandal-

H

ism; you certainly didn't get it in Paris — it's been raining non-stop.'

'Well, I did spend a couple of days in Cannes with a friend ... '

' ... where I gather from the weather report that it's been very sunny!'

'Oh yes, it was lovely! But I didn't go near the beach. We just wandered around.'

'And I suppose it didn't occur to you that the sun shines as much in the streets of Cannes, a few yards from the beach!'

'But we were in the car!'

'What sort of car? Was it open?'

'Yes ... '

So that was it!

'Didn't you realise what you were doing?'

'I used sun-screen cream, like you said.'

'What I said was that you must use sun-screen cream even though you were not to expose yourself to the sun on any pretext whatever for at least two months. The sun's destructive power is far greater than any resistance a sun-screen cream can offer. What's more, in an open car, the wind would have evaporated it and dried it up within an hour. You did precisely what I told you not to do: expose your skin to the sun without protection, with immediate consequences, no doubt.'

'It's true, it happened almost at once; within twenty-four hours. I'm absolutely desperate.'

The only time I ever hear this word it's in connection with some blemish which, however unsightly, is quite harmless: it doesn't form part of the vocabulary of the seriously ill. Perhaps the sheer weight of the word is meant to compensate for the trivial nature of the problem, the lack of any real cause for despair, and to arouse the interest and sympathy of the doctor.

However, she looked so miserable that I relented.

'We'll get rid of those marks of yours, but you won't be able to go out in the sun at all this summer; that's your punishment for being so careless.'

'Won't they go if I have another peeling?'

The properties of exfoliation

Certainly not! Freckles are the only kind of pigmentation which can be removed by peeling, because the melanin deposits are very superficial and confined to the horny layer. In the case of photo-sensitisation the pigmentation is too deep for exfoliation to be of any use.

It's exactly the same with chloasma, the facial pigmentation you sometimes get in pregnancy – peeling can't help there either, because the pigmentation is too deep. But whereas in chloasma exfoliation is merely ineffective, in cases where the pigmentation is caused through photosensitisation the remedy may be worse than the disease: a new application of phenol can revive or reinforce the allergic reaction.

On the whole, peeling isn't used to treat pigmentation marks; it's seldom effective and sometimes makes matters worse; even in the case of freckles its uses are very limited, because the freckles will reappear with the first rays of the sun in the same numbers and to the same degree as before.

On the other hand, peeling is a very useful and sometimes strikingly successful treatment for acne, scarring, certain congestive conditions that redden the skin, second-degree ageing and superficial lines.

How exfoliation works

Desquamation is far from being the most significant and important thing that happens in peeling. To put it another way, *the reason peeling is effective is not because it causes the skin to peel.*

The principal effects of exfoliation, which make it so valuable and more than simply a peeling of the skin, are to be found deep in the epidermis and in the dermis.

Effects on the epidermis

During exfoliation, the basal cells of the epidermis multiply profusely: the resulting production of young cells not only entails a rapid renewal of the basal layers of the epidermis but also an increase in their number. Consequently, after peeling, there is a thickening of the epidermis; and what is more to the point, this thickening applies to the layers of living cells.

Rejuvenation

Bearing in mind that the decrease in the number of layers of living cells and the increase in the number of layers of dead horny cells is one of the characteristics of ageing skin — whether due to the course of nature or to the sun — then peeling, by augmenting the former and diminishing the latter, restores the structures of the ageing epidermis to something resembling those of youthful skin. I dislike the term rejuvenation, because it has been so misused; nevertheless these effects constitute a genuine rejuvenation of the epidermal tissue.

Scars

In the same way, by causing the epidermal cells to multiply, peeling can improve the appearance of sunken scars such as the pits left by acne spots, especially when these have been exacerbated by picking or squeezing.

The epidermis is always thin over a scar (or 'atrophied', as I explained earlier). All scars, in fact, are the result of the destruction of the cells in the basal layer, the parent cells of all other epidermal cells. These cells do not regenerate themselves. Their loss being permanent, wounds can only be repaired by the undamaged basal cells on the perimeter of the destroyed zone; or else, if the zone is traversed by the duct from a sebaceous gland, by the cells which form its walls and which have the same properties as basal cells. In either case, the repair is never invisible, and, as the epidermis is abnormally thin over a wound, the scar forms a hollow. By increasing the thickness of the diminished epidermis, peeling helps to fill in the hollow. It will never disappear completely: anyone who expects his scars to vanish after peeling is doomed to disappointment. Only superficial scars can be improved and made nearly invisible. Pronounced scars are better treated by methods which I shall come to later.

Effects on the dermis

The cellular activity provoked by peeling isn't confined to the epidermis. The connective cells of the dermis multiply at the same rate and produce new bundles of fibrous tissue.

In an ageing dermis, one that is becoming thin and lax, this proliferation of cells amounts to a restoration: the dermis becomes denser, more compact and consequently firmer; in this case, it's much more than a repair, it's a renewal, leaving the skin improved in firmness and tone.

Furthermore, the arteries and veins in the dermis dilate, with the result that the treated zone receives an increased blood supply. This is why, incidentally, it reddens, burns and occasionally even swells a little during peeling.

This vascular response is important because, as we have seen, it is from the arterial blood that all living cells, including those of the skin, obtain the oxygen and nutrients essential to them; and by means of the venous blood that the carbon dioxide gas and the waste products of cellular 'digestion' are excreted.

I'm not telling the reader anything that he or she doesn't already know when I point out that someone who expends energy requires more sugars, fats and proteins – and uses up more oxygen – than someone who is sedentary

But an individual is no more than the sum of the thousands of millions of cells which go to make up his body, at which level the same process applies. Multiplying cells consume a great deal of energy, and without the increased blood supply that accompanies peeling they would be unable to proliferate. These phenomena – the multiplication of the cells of both epidermis and dermis and the stimulation of the local blood supply – are not mere guesswork, they have been confirmed by examination under the microscope of pieces of skin (biopsies) taken from volunteers throughout the exfoliation process. It has also been established that these effects continue for about three weeks after exfoliation is complete, that is, after the skin has ceased to peel. This means that the full benefit of peeling cannot be seen for about a month.

Clearly, all this activity, cellular and circulatory, is constructive and causes no weakening of the skin whatsoever. Quite the contrary, in fact; the skin emerges with new and lasting strength. In many cases the beneficial effects last for a year. Once this complex mechanism – a long way from most people's concept of 'stuff used to peel the skin' – has been understood, one can then understand:

1 Why the stimulation of the connective tissue makes it possible to reduce superficial wrinkles (deep lines, like deep scars, require other procedures);

2 Why the stimulation of the blood-vessels makes it possible to relieve certain congestive conditions of the face where there is diffuse redness of the skin from abnormal slowness of blood-flow in the tiny vessels of the dermis;

3 Why, at a time when there was no effective medication for

acne, peeling was of real value to some patients because of its deep action and the fact that, by unplugging the pores, it allowed the elimination of closed comedones and blackheads. In those days, it was the main treatment for acne. Today I regard it as the finishing touch, and I seldom have recourse to it except to restore the wear and tear of years of illness, once the acne has been cured;

4 Why peeling has no effect on normal skin. In a normal skin cellular reproduction is at its optimum; the fabric of the dermis could not be denser, the living cells more numerous or the horny layer thinner. To stimulate them would therefore be pointless: the normal skin peels very little during exfoliation and emerges exactly the same as it was before.

Exfoliation can be repeated at will. There's no limit to the number of peelings a skin will stand — which is not surprising, considering that each peeling stimulates regrowth.

Theoretically, one could even undertake several peelings one after the other, beginning again as soon as the previous one was completed, without the slightest risk. In practice, however, this is almost never done. Experience has shown that when two peelings are effected at two weeks' interval, that is when the cellular reproduction begun by the first has still not finished by the time one embarks on the second, one nearly always obtains markedly better results than would be the case had the same two peelings been undertaken two or three months apart. If two peelings seem advisable, because of the degree of skin damage to be treated, it would therefore seem best to arrange for them to be done in quick succession. The cumulative effect of peelings repeated at short intervals is particularly noticeable when treating facial redness.

That said, I must reiterate that peeling is not a cure-all. People who expect it to give them the skin of a new-born baby are doomed to disappointment and should be discouraged. You can't make calf's skin out of old tanned leather whatever you do. If the skin is to respond to the stimulation of peeling, it must be still capable of doing so. If it has become completely amorphous, peeling will have no effect. It is up to the dermatologist to judge, and, as often as not, he will advise against peeling, not because of any risk or other drawback involved, but simply because it wouldn't be worth it.

THIRD STAGE: THE SKIN IS DRIED UP, LAX, ATONIC AND DEEPLY LINED

In this case, the drying up of the horny layer and the atrophy of the dermis are accompanied by degeneration of the elastic tissue. The face has a worn look which in no way reflects the general physical condition. The upper eyelids droop like empty bags over the eyelashes; the lower lids form pockets which are sometimes accentuated by little cushions of fat; the skin sags into jowls along the jawline; wrinkles are no longer mere lines, but folds, or deep creases, on the forehead and between the eyebrows; at the outer corner of the eyes, the laughter lines have become 'crow's feet'; a cleft separates the cheek from the mouth which seems to recede between two flabby mounds of flesh.

The neck, too, becomes slack: instead of being held firmly in place by the special muscle attached to the innermost surface of the skin, which gave its shape and tension, it begins to hang loose like a turkey's wattle.

By this stage, it is not only the neck-muscle which has slackened; all the facial muscles lose their tension and add their effect to that of the other changes in the skin: all parts of the face show a tendency to droop in accordance with the laws of gravity; if the head is bent down they sag forwards, if tilted back, they slide backwards.

The face-lift

The answer is surgery. The slack in the skin must be taken up. In the three hours it takes to do a face-lift the surgeon can eradicate the traces of fifteen to twenty years of wear and tear. These days, the face-lift is a routine operation whose results are practically guaranteed. They depend entirely on the surgeon's touch and eye, on not taking up too much skin, or too little.

Its primary objective is to eradicate the wrinkles on the cheeks, chin and neck; in principle, it consists of detaching large areas of the skin of the cheeks and neck and tightening it by pulling it towards the ears in such a way as to remodel the facial contours, and finally, stitching up after the excess skin has been removed. The incisions are made in the crease between cheeks and ears, and behind the ears extending backwards into the hair.

There's no reason why the operation should not be done under

a local anaesthetic, but since it takes a long time, nervous patients
may require a general anaesthetic.

The first pressure dressing is left in place for forty-eight hours.
The patient can leave the hospital or nursing home after two or
three days. A certain amount of swelling will persist for a week.
Provided that the blood-vessels have been meticulously tied,
haematomas (the correct name for what we call bruises, caused by
bleeding under the skin) will not form. The stitches are removed
gradually between the fifth and tenth days after the operation.

The scars, in the shape of fine red lines, are visible for two or
three months, but women can easily conceal them by rearranging
their hair-style; they don't interfere with normal activity, which
may be resumed after ten days, or two weeks at most. Scars in
front of the ear gradually fade until they're totally invisible; behind
the ears and in the hair around the temples where one usually extends the incisions designed to efface the 'crow's feet', they will
always be somewhat enlarged.

This presents men with a problem: lifting is just as effective for
them as it is for women, but it's very difficult, if not impossible,
for a man to conceal these particular scars in his hair.

The face-lift is unquestionably the principal means of 'rejuvenating' the face. The improvement lasts for several years, five on
average; in the least favourable circumstances it may not last longer
than three years, but in the best cases it can last as long as ten.

When the skin begins to sag once again, the operation can be
repeated, and two face-lifts in a life-time is by no means unreason-
able; but it is most inadvisable to have more than three. The
quality and durability of the improvement depend to a large extent
on the patient's state of health and fluctuations in weight, as well
as on the climate (the effects of a face-lift are not as long-lasting in
hot countries), the shape of the face and the type of skin.

On a person over fifty, with an oval-shaped face and fine skin,
a face-lift is strikingly successful. People with square faces or
short necks make less suitable subjects. Obese people are doomed
to disappointment in that the hoped-for refinement of the features
cannot be achieved unless they first get down to something like
normal weight.

Seborrheic skin responds poorly to surgery, and in very dried-up
skins the effects tend to wear off fairly quickly.

It's in cases like these where medical treatments such as hormone creams and peeling still have their uses. Although inadequate by themselves as a remedy for the critical situation brought about by the destruction of the elastic tissues of the dermis, they still retain to some degree their effect on the dermal and epidermal structures. If, by this stage, they no longer constitute the treatment of choice for skin-ageing, they are nevertheless necessary and useful complements to surgery in that they can improve or prolong its effects. Hormone creams can still be used twice a day, for as long as is desired. Peeling can be done both before the operation, in order to give the surgeon the best possible material to work on, and afterwards, in order to postpone the day when a second operation is required.

Tightening the skin laterally and vertically at the ears and temples will correct the jowls, the folds in the cheeks on either side of the mouth, the 'crow's feet' and the neck-wattle; it will not correct the lines on the forehead, the bulges on the eyelids or, should this be pronounced, the cushion of fat which forms the so-called double chin.

Each of these particular types of progressive skin damage requires a special operation.

Eyelid surgery

Eyelid surgery is extremely simple because of the remarkable quality of the skin on the eyelids which always heals quickly and satisfactorily. The incisions, made immediately below the lashes on the lower lids and in the fold made by the eyeball on the upper lids, are easily and naturally concealed. All four eyelids can be treated in a single operation. The dressing is left in place for only twenty-four hours and the stitches are removed on the third or fourth day. Light make-up can be used after about ten days. Swelling is almost non-existent, so much so that with the help of a pair of tinted glasses the daily routine need hardly be interrupted.

The results are excellent and last considerably longer than the effects of a face-lift: indeed, they are virtually permanent. Eyelid surgery is equally successful in men, for whom the post-operative period and the disappearance of the scars take even less time than they do in women.

It can be a good idea to operate on the eyelids separately, before any face-lifting operation is required; when, for example, the eyelids are deformed by cushions of fat without showing other signs of ageing. By the time the facial skin is in need of lifting, the eye-lids will be in an equally critical condition – and wrinkled, droop-ing eyelids would be quite unacceptable in an otherwise smooth, taut face.

In other words, a face-lift necessarily implies eyelid surgery. But the two operations should not be done at the same time, as lifting will needlessly exaggerate the post-operative swelling of the eyelids which always suffer as a result. Consequently the eyelids are treated in a second operation, whereas lifting and surgery of a double chin can perfectly well be done at the same time as lifting and surgery of the lines of the forehead (known as frontal rid-ectomy).

Frontal ridectomy

This operation is performed either by making an incision from one ear to the other, hidden an inch or so behind the hairline, or by means of an incision which follows the line of the eyebrows and can be rectified later if need be. The skin on the forehead is com-pletely detached in order that not only the horizontal creases but also the vertical folds between the eyebrows may be eradicated. Some surgeons take away the frontal muscle: the removal of this muscle ensures the total and lasting disappearance of the lines, but it is not always desirable because a forehead that is too smooth and immobile lacks expression.

Apart from exceptional cases, none of these operations is justified in patients under the age of forty. Doctors frequently have either to talk their patients out of having surgery, or persuade them to wait until an operation is necessary, or even get them to renounce altogether measures which offer little hope of improvement.

Partial face-lift

The partial face-lift is a case in point. It seems to me a senseless procedure, not merely because the results are generally poor and short-lived, but also because, for the sake of harmony, the rejuven-ation of the features must be homogeneous: when one part of the face alone is improved, it accentuates the deterioration of the rest. It is far better to persuade the patient to put things off for two or three years and then do a complete face-lift.

Lifting at the temples only is a typical example of a partial face-lift. Sometimes known as 'mannequin's lift', it appeals to young women who imagine they need it because, when they smile, their skin creases slightly at the corner of their eyes. The vast majority soon realise, too late, that they've gained little, if any, benefit from it. As, indeed, was only to be expected.

Women who imagine that they are ageing prematurely make the ideal prey for the type of surgical practice which puts the operation before the patient. As a plastic surgeon, a friend of mine, wrote in 1968: 'To know when to operate is the be-all and end-all of surgical integrity; in cosmetic surgery, this extends to considerations of good taste and moderation.'

Such considerations preclude, among other things, agreeing to perform a face-lift on a thirty-year old woman, however much she insists on it by harping on the imperfections, more imaginary than real, that she fancies she has detected. A friend of mine once sent just such a girl to see me two days before she was due to have her operation. It would clearly have been madness, and I'm happy to say that I managed to persuade her to give up the idea.

On the other hand, similar considerations may prompt one to encourage those women to go ahead who, although deeply depressed by their appearance, are too apprehensive, or even, as is not uncommon at the menopause, too apathetic to take the plunge. It's very gratifying to see them after the operation, their attitude to life transformed together with the transformation of their features.

Wrinkles of the upper lip

The post-operative shock being negligible, it is no more difficult to do a face-lift on a woman of sixty than on a woman of forty. But a face-lift cannot deal with a defect common at the age of sixty: I refer to the lines on the upper lip which present a problem that is extremely difficult to solve.

These wrinkles are particularly unsightly, accentuated as they are with every contraction of the muscle surrounding the mouth, giving it a puckered look; and the more successful the face-lift, the more noticeable these lines become. Lifting has no effect on them because the traction of the skin only extends to the fold between the cheeks and mouth. To deal with them one must have recourse to different methods.

Personally, I'm strongly averse to the method whereby silicone is injected beneath the line of the wrinkle in order to try to bring it level with the surrounding skin. I've known this result in inflam-

mation, the formation of permanent hard fibrous nodules or re-
tractions, or even, in one case, death of the skin. The dermis tends
to reject foreign substances, and such reactions are unforeseeable.

There are only two methods of treatment which can be considered
valid, neither of them very pleasant: dermabrasion and peeling by
means of neat phenol.

Dermabrasion or skin-planing

Invented by an American, this method consists of 'planing' the
skin with metal brushes or grinding discs revolving at speed. They
are attached to an electrical hand-held apparatus, something like a
piece of dental equipment, requiring considerable skill to operate.
This appliance abrades the epidermis down to the level of the
dermis. In order to prevent the skin from being torn by the spin-
ning action of the discs, it is first frozen by a jet of liquid snow
which gives off intense cold by evaporation. This gives a hardened
surface to work on. The refrigeration also prevents the exposed
surface from bleeding too freely during the operation.

Dermabrasion not only makes it possible to treat the wrinkles of
the upper lip but also those scars which are too deep to respond
satisfactorily to peeling.

Some specialists use dermabrasion over the entire face. There is
no doubt that, when carried out by a skilled practitioner, it gives
excellent results where the face is badly pitted after severe acne.
It should be emphasised that before risking dermabrasion on a
patient who has had acne, the skin must be completely cured. In a
patient who still possesses closed comedones and pustules, dermabrasion is strictly contra-indicated. (Peeling, on the other hand
may safely be undertaken.)

On the whole, I am rather disillusioned with this technique, and
I know that many of my colleagues share my feelings. Post-operative care is protracted and difficult and the post-operative period
very long: the skin takes a good fortnight to heal and dressings are
essential throughout this period, as is a preventive course of antibiotics. The epidermis repairs itself through the cells of the
sebaceous duct.

One is left with a smooth surface of scar tissue which stays red
for several weeks. On average, it takes at least three if not four
months for the treated surface to fade and become white. Moreover, this whiteness is not that of normal skin: by destroying the

epidermal cells down to the basal layer, the pigment cells have also been destroyed. This is unavoidable. In fact, as I shall explain later, this destruction is used to treat pigmentation marks caused by the sun (so-called 'senile' pigmentation). Once an area has been treated by dermabrasion it never again produces pigment and will always have the same white, rather nacreous appearance which is characteristic of all cutaneous scars whatever their origin. Patients should be warned that this is the price they will have to pay for getting rid of the wrinkles on their upper lip.

Furthermore, I believe you need to be strongly motivated to accept all the constraints involved, just as you must be to accept those which result from peeling with pure phenol.

Peeling with pure phenol

I should point out at once that this is not the same type of exfoliation as that I mentioned when describing Unna's method: in this case complete destruction of the epidermis is involved.

In addition, when using pure phenol in the treatment of scars, one must leave an interval of at least two to three months before repeating a treatment, and it may be repeated only two or three times. One can immediately see that it is very different from resorcin exfoliation, which can safely be repeated once every week if you so wish. In fact it amounts to chemical, rather than mechanical dermabrasion, or what the Americans call 'chemosurgery'. Over large surfaces its use is both impracticable and dangerous.

For wrinkles on the upper lip, the recommended method is to cover the zone treated with phenol with adhesive plaster strips so that the destroyed epidermis comes away as these are torn off. As in dermabrasion, the dermis is then exposed. Because of the toxicity of phenol, which forbids its use on patients with a history of kidney trouble, some specialists prefer to use 50 per cent aqueous trichloracetic acid.

This acts in the same way as phenol; to call the treatment trichloracetic acid exfoliation, however, is again incorrect. Like phenol, trichloracetic acid provokes a chemical dermabrasion and not an exfoliation.

The application is frankly painful and entails the same postoperative risks of white, permanently depigmented skin as dermabrasion, or else of brownish patches, especially around the edges of treated surfaces.

I'm told that in the United States certain dermatologists and cosmetic surgeons don't hesitate to use this treatment on the eyelids, and that their patients agree to submit to it. I only hope that these men are well-insured, considering how quick Americans are to sue their doctors on the slightest pretext!

Although I'm a strong supporter of cosmetic surgery in skilled and experienced hands, I have equally strong reservations about such drastic methods, because they entail too high a risk of unforeseeable accidents. It's all very well to say: *il faut souffrir pour être belle*, but you should think long and hard before you risk being permanently disfigured!

TABLE II Summary of treatments involving skin ageing according to the degree of severity

	Protective cream water-in-oil emulsion	Water-in-oil emulsion cream + hormones	Peeling	Cosmetic surgery	Dermabrasion Mechanical	Chemical
1st stage: dried-up skin (rough skin)	Yes (day and night)	No	No	No	No	No
2nd stage: rough skin, thickening of horny layer of the epidermis, dermis loses resilience (atrophic)	No	Yes (day and night)	Yes (treatment of choice)	No	No	No
3rd stage: rough, lined skin, thickened horny layer, atrophic, atonic dermis	No	Yes (day and night)	Yes to complement surgery	Yes (face-lift and eyelid surgery [treatment of choice] frontal ridectomy; double chin)	With reservations (upper lip)	No (upper lip)

4 Other important changes affecting the skin

The skin of every human being, regardless of sex or origin, goes through the different stages I have just described. These may occur early or late, quickly or slowly, completely or partially, depending on the colour of your skin, how you look after it, your professional occupation, the extent to which this exposes you to the rigours of climate and the amount of sunshine in the country where you live.

Yet the various types of progressive skin damage in the dermis and epidermis associated with the process of ageing, whether natural and delayed or artificial and premature, are far from being the only such changes the skin is heir to.

Whereas none of us can escape senile degeneration to some degree, there are other important changes of the skin which should be dealt with separately because they have certain distinctive characteristics and respond to specific methods of treatment. That is why I have decided to devote this chapter to them.

Some, of course, are part of the process of ageing: by which I mean that they would not exist were the skin not senescent; not that these disorders – the 'solar' or 'senile' lentiginoses and keratoses to which I referred earlier in the section on ageing skin, and seborrheic warts – need necessarily be present in an ageing skin.

Others are independent of the ageing process and can occur as easily in young people as in their elders: these are the pigmentary disorders, circulatory disorders, disorders of the elastic tissue and disorders associated with sweating and abnormal hair-growth.

CHANGES ASSOCIATED WITH AGEING SKIN
'SOLAR' LENTIGINOSES

The despair of middle-aged women, who know only too well what they portend, 'solar' or 'senile' lentiginoses are very common. After the age of fifty they appear in one person in every three, men as well as women.

They are darkish brown, quite flat and persist indefinitely;

once formed, their colour is not affected by exposure to the sun.

They occur mostly on the back of the hands, where I have seen them in such quantities that they covered the hands completely in one uniform mass. They can also occur on the face and the V-shaped area at the base of the neck.

Their treatment is simple.

One can use either carbon dioxide snow, liquid nitrogen or electrocoagulation.

Unlike carbon dioxide snow and liquid nitrogen, which coagulate the cutaneous cells by cold, electrocoagulation does so by the heat of an electric spark produced by a high-frequency alternating generator. The heat and strength of the spark can be regulated on this type of apparatus; in the case in point, fine needles and a weak current are used.

These procedures are a little lacking in precision in that there is a risk, even for the experienced operator, of coagulating very slightly more than necessary.

I therefore prefer the dermabrasion technique, using very small discs, which allows one to see exactly what one is doing and to limit the abrading to what is strictly necessary. With unduly sensitive or nervous patients there's no harm in using a local anaesthetic, but the operation is not unpleasant and can easily be done without anaesthetic. Bleeding is slight; a scab forms which becomes detached after a week, as with any ordinary superficial graze.

The only drawback common to all types of dermabrasion, is that the reconstituted skin is rather whiter than normal, at least for some time. But exactly the same applies to coagulation, and, in any event, a faint white mark is much less noticeable than a dark brown one.

This superficial and purely cosmetic treatment, when delicately done, entails only one risk: that, due to the operator's lightness of touch, the lentiginoses will not disappear completely. But this is a fault on the right side, and with such wholly benign pigmentations the worst that can happen is that one may have to do a little retouching, which is neither serious nor complicated.

PRE-CANCEROUS MELANOSIS

The same cannot be said of certain pigmented marks on the face which should be treated with the utmost caution because, while

I

somewhat resembling lentiginoses, these lesions are in reality potential cancers.

Unlike 'senile' lentiginoses, pre-cancerous melanosis can appear at any age — 50 per cent of cases occur before the age of forty. It also differs in that the lesion is not uniform in colour: some areas are lighter than others. Lastly, it has a tendency to spread gradually, like a grease-spot; some lesions have been known to reach the size of the palm of the hand.

Not only is it an unsightly lesion, it's a dangerous one; in 50 per cent of cases, it will develop into cancer. This development is signalled by the appearance in the pigmented area of extrusions something like warts, or rough surface scabs on surfaces hitherto smooth to the touch. These should be destroyed by electro-coagulation, as in the case of lentiginoses, but at greater strength and much greater depth. However, the malignancy* of these cancers is fortunately not very great, and, in their case, partial destruction is adequate, *whereas in the case of cancer of a certain type of mole or beauty-spot, which I shall come to in a moment, such limited destruction is literally a crime.*

SEBORRHEIC WARTS

The same methods of treatment, with the same results, may be applied to the ugly formations known as seborrheic or 'senile' warts.

These lesions, found in both sexes, are as common as they are innocuous and benign: they are oval-shaped extrusions, covered in very greasy squames, more or less perched on the surface of the skin; their colour varies from grey to dark brown, some being almost black.

Unlike lentiginoses and keratoses, the sun plays no part in their development, with the result that some skins are entirely free from them.

Seborrheic warts appear in crops from middle age onwards, usually on the torso, less often on the neck, face or scalp. Sometimes there are just a few, sometimes hundreds. They develop and gradually enlarge over an indefinite period: I remember once destroying one as big as a saucer. There is everything to be gained

---

* Malignancy means the potential behaviour and progress of a cancer. Cancer and malignant tumour are synonymous. (A-B)

by treating them while they are still small. The destruction of one
seborrheic wart does not, of course, mean that others will not
appear elsewhere; and there is no preventive treatment one can
apply to them. But at least destruction in the early stages means
that they won't grow to any size and their treatment is thus greatly
simplified: it is obviously easier to remove a small lesion than a
large one, and the smaller it is, the quicker it will heal.

Where the treatment of cosmetic disorders is concerned, there
is never any point in putting off until tomorrow what can be done
today.

'SOLAR' KERATOSES

Lesions of this type are a very different matter: 'senile' or 'solar'
keratoses occur exclusively in those areas exposed to sunlight
(mainly the face and the back of the hands) and, as we have seen
they constitute pre-cancerous lesions.* Beware of any brownish-red
mark that begins to feel rough to the touch: true, by no means all
such lesions will necessarily become cancers, but one can never be
sure that one or more of them will not develop in this direction at
some time or other. It is far better not to wait for this eventuality,
especially when they occur on the scalp of a bald man, where they
are very common, or on the ears: although skin cancers are much
less malignant than internal cancers as a general rule, being
simpler to destroy and nearly always completely curable, those on
the scalp and ears are infinitely more serious and resistant to
treatment.

In such cases, therefore, the rule I have just stated, never pro-
crastinate, applies with even greater force.

In its early stages the lesion can be treated economically, so to
speak, that is without destroying too wide or too deep an area; it
is sufficient to use either electrocoagulation or coagulation by
means of cold, at hardly greater strength than that required in the
case of seborrheic warts or lentiginoses.

Dermabrasion may even be used, followed by a brief application
of trichloracetic acid which chemically coagulates the exposed surface of the dermis and gives additional protection.

But if there is any suspicion of malignant change, manifested
by a tendency of the lesion to protrude, and especially if it shows

* A description of this lesion also appears on p. 68. (Tr)

signs of growing inwards and ulcerating, it must be completely destroyed with electric cautery.

In this sun-worshipping age, keratoses are becoming more and more common, and the number of people affected is increasing all the time. The punishment for past carelessness, they sprout up over the years, one after another, now on the nose, now on the ears and forehead; once they have begun to appear, it is quite probable that you will have to have them removed at intervals for the rest of your life.

It's not merely a question of looks: *the treatment of keratoses the moment they appear is tantamount to preventing cancer.*

CHANGES INDEPENDENT OF AGEING SKIN

These are extremely varied and can affect skin colour, circulation and the hair, as well as the dermis and hypodermis.

PIGMENTARY DISORDERS

I have already referred in passing to ephelids or freckles and also to pigmentation from perfumes, in particular bergamot oil, due to sun sensitivity or photosensitisation. It seems unnecessary, therefore, to repeat myself here.

Particularly as the former are not really considered to be blemishes: there's nothing displeasing about a pretty redhead with a face dusted with freckles. As for the phenomenon of sensitivity, it is easily avoided: you only have to be careful never to use scented products before sun-bathing.

It's a very different matter when we come to consider two other forms of abnormal pigmentation, one, chloasma, caused by an excess of pigment, the other, vitiligo, by a lack of it.

No one really knows the underlying causes of these two conditions, which have in common their unattractiveness, their stubborn resistance to treatment, but, happily, their otherwise total harmlessness.

CHLOASMA

Chloasma is a dirty-grey, rather than brown, pigmentation, which very occasionally appears on the breasts and in the genital region but which usually occurs on the face, where it takes on a character-istic pattern: a broad vertical band of pigment appears in the middle of the forehead and divides to follow the line of the eye-brows; below this there are usually a few patches of pigment on the tip of the nose, a pigmented band across the upper lip like a moustache and, less frequently, another on the point of the chin. The band over the eyebrows occasionally extends to encircle the eyes, following the line of the eye-sockets. If the cheeks are affected, the pigmentation takes the form of a rough triangle with the point facing towards the nose.

Between these expanses of pigment the skin colour is normal. The more the pigmentation changes colour, the more unsightly the effect: it fades in winter until it is hardly distinguishable from normal skin except in a certain light, and darkens with the sun in summer.

The commonest and oldest-known cause of chloasma, some-times called the 'mask of Venus', is pregnancy, during which it can occur at any stage, early or late, often disappearing soon after delivery. Unfortunately, however, it sometimes persists for months or years, or even indefinitely.

But pregnancy isn't the only cause of chloasma: it has been known to appear during the development of cancer of the digestive tract; it can occur in women with diseases of the uterus or the ovaries, or even, lacking any organic cause whatever, in people suffering from emotional shock, nervous tension or depression. Few people realise that it can also occur in men.

However, by far the most frequent cause of chloasma these days is the pill: all types of contraceptive pill, even the weaker kind we call mini-pills, can cause this troublesome pigmentation. Neverthe-less, this reaction always demands sunlight: as long as the face is not exposed to the sun, nothing happens. In fact, the frequency of chloasma in women on the pill is much greater in sunny coun-tries: only about 5 per cent of Frenchwomen are affected, compared with 45 per cent of Puerto Rican women, for instance.

Some people think that women on the pill should be advised not to take it during the summer months. The idea has met with little enthusiasm: the summer holidays are hardly the time to advocate sexual restraint, and, in any case, this would simply be to replace one risk by another, more serious one; women who take the pill are, by definition, women who don't want to get pregnant, and a

woman with an unwanted pregnancy will do anything to rid herself of it, even to the point of risking her life.

Incidentally, I've always been struck by the way in which a
woman who is sufficiently determined not to have a baby will put
up with her chloasma rather than give up the pill: naturally, she
dislikes it, but she accepts it without fuss. Even when she asks for
advice, more often than not she will neglect to follow it properly,
if at all.

This behaviour is in marked contrast to that of women whose
chloasma springs from other causes; for example, when it persists
after pregnancy. Such women show a fierce determination to be
cured and stick to the treatment — which is extremely slow in producing any response — in the face of all discouragement.

The fact is that although we know the circumstances which may
give rise to chloasma, we know nothing, as I hinted at the beginning of this chapter, about its underlying causes.

Why is it, for example, that the same cause will not always produce the same effect? The majority of pregnant women never
suffer from chloasma, and other women will get it after having
come through two or three pregnancies unscathed. What is the
reason for the characteristic pattern of the pigmentation, which
leaves whole areas of the skin unaffected? These questions remain
unanswered. There is some reason to believe that this disorder is
influenced by hormones and the central nervous system. But precisely how is yet another question mark.

Nor, in the fog surrounding this problem, do we have a valid
internal treatment to offer; we have to do the best we can with
external applications. These contain a substance used in the photo-
graphic and rubber-processing industries which has the property
of removing the pigment from normal skin. Indeed, it was through
observing the discoloration on the hands of workers in synthetic
rubber factories that this property was first discovered.

The parent substance, hydroquinone, requires careful handling,
since it can cause photosensitisation. There is a chemical derivative
available in the form of an ointment which is less allergy-provoking
but also less active.* It has to be applied daily over a period of
months, if not longer, and care must be taken not to let it come
into contact with the healthy skin which is much more easily dis-

* It has been shown recently that the effect of hydroquinone can be improved
by the addition of Retinoic acid to the ointment. (A-B)

coloured than the affected part. Above all, the face must not be exposed to the sun during treatment or there is a danger of losing in a single day what it has taken months to achieve: chloasma darkens in the sun with remarkable speed and intensity.

A sunshade, a wide-brimmed hat and a thick screen of protective cream are the indispensable adjuncts to this irksome treatment which must be carried out with the utmost punctiliousness. Indeed, it should only be undertaken on the clear understanding that patience and perseverance are the *sine qua non* of success.

For the time being, unfortunately, there is no other treatment. As I explained earlier, peeling has no effect on chloasma: I emphasise this yet again, because many people think that it has. Not only is it ineffective, but it often makes the condition worse due to the photosensitising effects of exfoliant preparations.

VITILIGO

In a sense, this justly dreaded complaint is the reverse of chloasma. Instead of the pigment accumulating, it vanishes altogether, leaving patches of matt white skin, some large, some small, which stand out all the more because the surrounding skin colour is darker than normal: it's as though the pigment, forced out of the discoloured area, had accumulated around the edges instead.

Its discoloration apart, the structure of the affected skin presents no other anomalies. Vitiligo can occur anywhere on the body, on the torso and limbs as well as on the face and scalp. If a hairy region is affected the hair may turn white, but this is not always the case.

Vitiligo can occur at any age. It often appears for the first time after exposure to the sun. In any case the white patches always look more pronounced in summer due to the contrast with the brown healthy skin surrounding them. Unless treated, vitiligo lasts for life, either remaining static or slowly getting worse as the de-pigmented areas multiply and enlarge. It is sufficiently common for people to panic at the first sign of a patch of white skin.

However, vitiligo isn't the only cause of skin discoloration. Another cause, increasingly prevalent in these days of crowded bathing on beaches and in public swimming-baths, goes by the charming name of *pityriasis versicolor*. This is a microscopic yeast-like organism which can infest large areas of the surface of the skin. To the untrained eye the resulting depigmentation can look like vitiligo; but there is no darker outline and a characteristic squame can be detected if the epidermis is scratched with a finger-nail.

Rough, 'floury' patches of skin can also become depigmented: frequently seen on the face and shoulders of young women and children, they can easily be distinguished from vitiligo by their bran-like surface and their blurred outlines. They are bacterial in origin and encouraged by a chapped skin. And, here again, one often finds that hygienic products, containing either too much detergent or too strong a detergent for the skin in question, have been used.

I've never been able to understand, incidentally, why some mothers insist on scrubbing their children's faces and washing their hair in the same soap they use for their bodies. For one thing, the children detest it and it makes them cry, and, for another, this deplorable practice is harmful to the facial skin which, as I've repeatedly emphasised, is particularly vulnerable. It's sheer madness to use detergents which continually threaten its equilibrium by causing it to become chapped and dried up.

To return to vitiligo: its underlying causes are no better known than those of chloasma. Like chloasma, they may be associated with the hormonal and nervous systems, but this has yet to be proved; the treatment is consequently empirical.

It consists of taking in tablet form* or else painting on to the discoloured skin an extract derived from an Egyptian plant called *ammi majus*. If one then exposes the skin to natural sunlight or artificial ultra-violet rays,† the *ammi majus* will act as a photosensitiser and restore colour to the depigmented areas.

But it is such a powerful photosensitiser that it can be dangerous. The duration of the exposures must be very carefully timed. If these times are exceeded, severe burns may result. After exposure the skin must be carefully protected from any additional radiation; this is easy enough in the case of areas normally protected by clothing, but much more difficult in the case of the face and hands.

In fact, it's a fairly risky treatment hedged about with do's and don'ts: patients are never sufficiently warned of the need for precautions. Personally, I am always reluctant to advise it, especially

* *Psoralens*. (Tr)
† Or so-called 'black light'. (Tr)

as the results are rather unpredictable. For this reason it seems to me a sensible principle to keep it in reserve for those cases where the condition is particularly disfiguring and has serious repercussions on the patient's morale.

Where the lesions are extremely widespread, with a greater proportion of discoloured skin than healthy skin, it is preferable to attempt to 'bleach' the latter with hydroquinone derivatives than to restore the colour of the former by using *ammi majus* extract. I once succeeded in doing this for a young girl who had the worst vitiligo I have ever seen. She was also very 'disturbed', she 'had problems', as they say. She later found the man of her dreams and married him: at which point her vitiligo disappeared spontaneously and completely! This goes to show that there are always exceptions to every rule and that this supposedly incurable disease can, on occasion, clear up of its own accord.

NAEVI

Before leaving the subject of pigmentary disorders, I think it would be helpful to add a short digression on 'junctional naevi' or moles, more commonly known as beauty-spots. They are rather on the fringe of our subject since, strictly speaking, they don't constitute a deterioration of the skin. They should rather be considered as malformations which are either congenital, that is present from birth, or appear later in life. As a rule, they are black with accumulated pigment, but they can also be hardly coloured at all, or even quite colourless.

Some are no larger than blackheads, while others are huge, covering the back and shoulders like a cape, or the loins and buttocks like a pair of underpants, or even half the body. They may be flat, level with the surface of the skin, or they may protrude, when they are sometimes confused with so-called 'soft warts'. This confusion is all the more unfortunate since if you are misguided enough to try to squeeze an ordinary wart you won't do any grave harm,* whereas if you treat a mole or beauty-spot in the same way you court mortal danger, especially those found on the

---

* The worst that can happen is that it will give birth to other warts, and I take this opportunity of warning people that if they treat their own warts with silver nitrate, they will only succeed in causing half a dozen to appear where there was only one before. (A-B)

extremities: the worst are those on the feet and those which develop beneath the nails. Malignant change of a mole or beauty-spot is a very serious matter *which requires immediate medical attention.* Malignant melanoma, as this type of cancer is known, is capable of killing within three months. Cases where sufferers have survived for more than ten years are noted exceptions.

This tumour can be extraordinarily deceptive. You operate; all seems well for a year, two years, sometimes longer; then, quite suddenly, from no known starting-point, the tiger you thought you had appeased suddenly re-awakens. Crops of new tumours erupt on the skin at points far removed from the original lesion, as well as in the lungs and brain; the end comes within a few weeks.

It is the most painful diagnosis I ever have to make, especially when, as is often the case, the victim is young. An old person's death is part of the natural order of things; that of a young person is shocking. He stands there before you, brimful of life and health, unaware of the significance of his sinister little black bud; and you think to yourself: 'he's done for'; his only chance would have been to get proper advice the moment the first symptoms appeared, when the mole or beauty-spot had first begun to tingle and enlarge slightly.

Instead he waited for three to four months before seeing a doctor, and he even squeezed it a little to see if anything came out! Warning people about this is like beating your head against a brick wall. You might as well put a bullet through your brain as squeeze a mole or beauty-spot which has begun to alter in character – the only difference is that the result is not quite as instantaneous. Why do people have this appalling habit of picking at anything that protrudes from the skin? If you pick at a seborrheic wart, it doesn't matter very much; but in the case of a naevus the consequences could be terrifying. The trouble is that the layman cannot distinguish between the two. When in doubt leave well alone, touch nothing and go and see your doctor at once; don't put it off: postponing matters will only make them worse. Where is the sense in that? If it's 'nothing', you can please yourself whether or not to have treatment; but if it's 'something', then an early diagnosis means that all the odds are in your favour.

The inflexible rule is never to squeeze or pick at a mole or beauty-spot. People are at last becoming aware of this, but it cannot be repeated too often.

This doesn't mean that a naevus should never be touched at all; indeed, there are some cases where it is essential to operate preventively: when there's a risk of repeated irritation from shaving in the case of men, for instance, or from rubbing against a glove or a bra in the case of women. Even more important, if a naevus shows signs of rapid growth during pregnancy, or if it has been cut or scratched, the operation must be performed without delay. And it's also justified if the size or number of the naevi amounts to a disfigurement.

In France, the usual method is electrocoagulation. In America, surgery is preferred. In fact, one decides on the best method for each individual case. Electrocoagulation leaves an atrophic scar, but certain naevi can be removed by this method with hardly a trace. If the naevus is enlarged, on the other hand, or in a place where the stitches can be disguised by a natural fold in the skin, electric cautery — sometimes accompanied by a skin-graft — is the better method to use.

The important thing is that it should be completely destroyed: a properly destroyed naevus is quite harmless because it no longer exists.

DISORDERS OF THE CIRCULATION

CHRONIC REDNESS* AND BROKEN VEINS† OF THE FACE

After this long digression, I now return to true degenerative changes, in which, however, the sun, rather than age, plays the all-important role.

Chronic redness of the face and the blotchiness caused by broken veins are different degrees of the same malady.

Facial redness can be present from childhood. It involves no modification in either the texture or surface of the skin, which is a diffuse, rather bright red. This can become exaggerated by eating, emotion, or variations in temperature, to the point where it can turn purple and burn. It is commoner in girls, but boys can also suffer from it.

The minute blood-vessels of the dermis — the capillaries —

* A condition which used to be called *erythrose*. (Tr)
† The medical term for this condition is *telangiectasia*. (Tr)

dilate from the effect of unrelieved congestion until they gradually become visible as a network of lines of varying width. The finer the skin, the more noticeable they are: these are the so-called 'broken veins'. Their incidence has nothing to do with the quality of the skin: one finds broken veins in seborrheic skin, normal skin and dried-up skin.

There are good grounds for supposing that chronic redness of the cheeks is a congenital abnormality: since the same condition is often to be found in the parents or grandparents, *there would seem to be a predisposition to facial redness from birth*.

The reason why the redness is essentially confined to the cheeks, rarely developing on the nose and cheek-bones, is thought to be connected with the fact that the circulation of the blood in the vessels of the skin depends on the activity of the underlying muscles. Each muscular contraction acts as a pump and propels the blood into the part of the dermis immediately above the muscles. When these muscles are more or less immobile the blood tends to stagnate like water in a pond instead of flowing like water in a river. The area of the cheeks happens to be a particularly immobile one; unless we contort the muscles in a grimace, they seldom move. In people already predisposed, therefore, the ideal conditions exist for a state of permanent congestion.

This highly susceptible congestive state can be affected in varying degrees by a number of different factors.

THE ROLE OF DIGESTIVE DISORDERS

For example, it is affected by digestive disorders, although not the ones that usually come to mind, such as malfunction of the intestine or the liver.

Poor liver! It has been blamed for everything under the sun since time began: 1800 years ago, when Babylonian civilisation had spread throughout the Near East, people believed that the liver was the guardian of both life and soul.

The fact is that the liver has nothing whatsoever to do with facial redness, any more than with acne or eczema. But you sometimes have to waste a lot of breath, and sometimes even do tests to prove it, before people will believe you. Nor do people with broken veins suffer more from constipation than anyone else; as often as not, their bowels work perfectly normally. And I've yet to come across a single case where either dieting, no matter how strict, or laxative treatment has been of help. That is not to say that digestive disorders, or eating and drinking to excess, do not affect the progress of the disease, but they are only significant in so far as they are contributory causes of skin trouble.

Medically speaking, the causes of disease fall into three categories: constitutional, contributory and precipitating.

Constitutional causes are those which must be present in order for the disease to develop in the first place; at the beginning of this book we saw how the male hormone is the constitutional cause of seborrhea; and we have just seen how a congenital predisposition is the constitutional cause of chronic redness of the cheeks.

THE ROLE OF FOOD

Contributory causes are those which affect the progress of the disease, but only when the latter exists. For example, eating too much, or eating spicy, indigestible food can cause the redness of the cheeks to become temporarily worse after a meal. But this is only an exaggeration of a normal phenomenon: everyone suffers a reflex dilation of the vessels of the facial skin following the absorption of food of any kind. This doesn't show in people with matt complexions, but in someone with a flushed complexion, whose vessels are already dilated, any additional dilation is easily noticeable.

For this reason, it can help to be careful how you eat. Let me be quite clear: I'm not talking about dieting in the ordinary sense, because the nature of the food is of secondary importance. It's the quantity which matters above all; provided that they eat slowly and a little at a time, people suffering from facial redness can eat what they like.

Emotional upsets and nervous tension can also cause the face to flush, and in women who still have their periods, the female hormone has the property of dilating the capillary vessels. That's why there is often increased flushing at certain times during the menstrual cycle.

THE ROLE OF THE SUN

Precipitating factors are those which bring about a progressive and permanent worsening of the disease. Medicines containing the female hormone come into this category and are consequently not advisable in the case of people affected by red cheeks or broken veins.

But for people suffering from chronic redness of the face the chief enemy is, yet again, the sun. It is the sun which causes their condition to be complicated by broken veins and encourages the visible capillaries to enlarge and multiply. Wind, cold, heat and damp are notoriously bad for the skin; but they are less harmful than the sun. It goes without saying that at the first sign of reddening, the face should be rigorously protected from the sun.

THE TREATMENT OF FACIAL REDNESS

As long as there is no network of broken veins, the redness can be treated with carbon dioxide snow. This demands a certain skill if the treated area is not to be left too white; personally, I'm in favour of retaining a slight pinkness which gives the same effect as rouge and at the same time does away with the necessity for it.

THE TREATMENT OF BROKEN VEINS

Once there is a visible network of broken veins the best treatment consists of cauterising them by means of electrolysis or fine electro-coagulation: the needle is inserted every two or three millimetres or so, following the lines of the network. The more that can be done at a time, the better and quicker the result. Although not exactly painful, the sensation is fairly disagreeable and tickles horribly, especially in the nostrils.

Depending on the length of the session, the face will be a little swollen for between two and five days, and the minute scabs which form over each point of insertion will disappear within eight to ten days. On no account should they be picked off.

With a co-operative patient, four sessions should be enough, even in a really bad case, particularly when there's no necessity to repeat them at close intervals: one about every six weeks is ideal; this makes it possible to see clearly what has been done and what remains to be done.

ROSACEA

At best, congestive phenomena of the face are limited to chronic redness of the cheeks, whether or not aggravated by broken veins.

But for the unlucky few, further complications in the form of spots which thrive in these particular conditions can ensue. These spots can be either minute pimples the size of a pinhead, occasionally having a tiny white 'head', or much larger purplish lumps lying beneath the surface of the skin. Both kinds appear in a series of sudden outbreaks and may be accompanied by tingling or itching. This condition is popularly known as 'acne rosacea', a term which is not only deplorably inexact — *since it bears no relationship whatsoever to acne* — but can also lead to confusion when it comes to treatment.

Indeed, I often see people who have been using sulphur cream, tincture of iodine or strong antiseptics for weeks on end, with nothing to show for it, poor things, but an intense irritation of their extremely easily inflamed spots. I've already explained why this kind of treatment should not be used in cases of true acne. In so-called acne rosacea it causes absolute havoc.

As for the hormonal treatments which can be used in acne, these are completely ineffective in rosacea.

Remembering that every acne spot requires a closed comedone in order to develop, it follows that a spot without its closed comedone is not an acne spot.

Rosacea spots are not acne spots but what we call folliculitus, because they arise from the hair-follicle (I shall describe the hair-follicle in a later section on hirsutism).

If you lance one of these spots, large or small, and then press it, it will produce a tiny amount of colourless fluid or else a drop of whitish substance which is not, however, pus: the microbes it contains — more often than not it doesn't even contain any — are quite harmless. And never, under any circumstances, will you find closed comedones in rosacea spots.

In 1951 I suggested that these spots were allergic in origin, and went on to show that they could be cured by antibiotics. The allergic nature of rosacea has since been widely confirmed.* Nearly always it proves to be an allergy to one of the many microbes we all harbour in our intestines, throat, nose and mouth. In general, they co-exist happily with us. Those in the intestine even work to our advantage by producing part of the vitamin B_2 we all require. Occasionally, however, things go wrong; and the deterioration of

* This might be disputed by some British dermatologists. (Tr)

our relationship as hosts to these guests can take the form of an infection or, sometimes, an allergy.

In the case of an infection, a boil, for example, the hitherto harmless microbe turns nasty, attacks and attempts to destroy our cells. Our forces counter-attack by sending in squads of white blood corpuscles to the threatened spot. These encircle the enemy, the defenders suffer casualties, and it is their corpses which form the pus.

In the case of an allergy, the situation is quite different: the microbe responsible is not found in the spots themselves — which is why antiseptic preparations applied locally have no effect — but can lie passively anywhere in the organism; and in this case it's the organism which suddenly decides, one day, that it cannot put up with its presence any longer; we say that it has become intolerant. We are intolerant to strawberries in strawberry rash, to lipstick in lipstick eczema, to pollen in pollen asthma. In rosacea we are intolerant to a microbe, and any microbe can cause rosacea.

However, it can happen that the same microbe is responsible for both allergy and infection. If so, it's a stroke of luck, for it enables us to track it down. Thus, if you find and treat, say, chronic appendicitis, sinusitis, tonsillitis or a dental abscess, you clear everything up at once: the infection because the focus has been removed, and the allergic reaction of the skin because it was triggered by the microbes in the focus of infection.

Cases of rosacea linked to an infection of the tonsils, sinuses or appendix are not very common. Those associated with a dental infection, on the other hand, are more frequent than might be supposed. Foci of infection in the teeth are extraordinarily difficult to detect, especially when they are painless. The abscesses responsible, which develop at the root of a carious tooth, in the surrounding bone, most often occur after the nerve of the tooth has been killed, when the dental canal has not been properly stopped; and they can only be detected by X-rays. One can make some alarming discoveries in the form of badly-filled teeth and abscesses when one X-rays a patient with rosacea. Once an abscess has formed, it won't clear up until the tooth has been re-opened, treated, disinfected and properly re-filled. And all the time it's there, it is pouring its poisons into the system.

These dental lesions are a heart-specialist's nightmare because, in patients with valvular diseases of the heart, they can cause endocarditis; the seriousness of this complication—it was invariably fatal until the introduction of penicillin, but can be cured these days by the injection of between 50 and 100 million units of penicillin a day over a period of weeks—gives some idea of the importance of sources of infection in the teeth.

Clearly, rosacea arising from a source of this kind will be incurable and resist all forms of treatment as long as the teeth are not properly looked after.

Here is one, absolutely typical, example:

Mrs P. is a hairdresser by profession and owns a salon in a country town. When she told me her story she was forty years old.

She developed rosacea at the age of thirty-six. She had no other symptoms which might have explained it: she had never had tonsillitis or sinusitis, and she didn't have toothache—she told me that her teeth were well cared-for; her bowels worked well and she wasn't constipated. She had never had a genital or urinary infection; she had never had a miscarriage and her only child, a son, was eighteen years old. Her periods were regular and quite normal, without headaches or pain or swelling of the breasts; if anything, they were slight, which meant nothing, and of short duration; she had no bleeding during ovulation.

She had had hundreds of injections of vitamin B_2, in vain, having been told that they would improve her rosacea—true enough, if you're content with very little improvement.

Colleagues who had seen her before she came to me had prescribed large doses over a two-month period of the drug used to treat the yeast responsible for thrush in suckling infants, familiar to nursing mothers, which can sometimes cause rosacea in adults. Following that, she had taken seven to eight capsules of Chloromycetin a day for several weeks. (Chloromycetin is the antibiotic most effective in rosacea: through it, twenty years ago, I discovered that this hitherto virtually incurable disease could be treated by this type of antibiotic, with spectacular results; in the majority of cases the eruption cleared up in three to four days; moreover a very weak dose, three to four capsules a day, was sufficient.)

Listening to her, I thought to myself that she was lucky that nothing had gone wrong: in fact, Chloromycetin is no longer prescribed for rosacea because it has been shown to destroy bone-marrow, with possibly fatal consequences. While one might be prepared to take the risk in the case of severe illness, it is un-

K

thinkable to do so in the case of a disease which, however unsightly, distressing and even unendurable in its tenacity, is nevertheless benign.

Moreover, there are now alternative antibiotics, such as the Tetracyclines, which my patient had also been taking, more or less continuously, in doses of six to eight capsules a day, or twice as much as is needed to clear up the spots in straightforward rosacea.

On top of all this, morning and night for four years she had been using an ointment on her face containing a very active cortisone derivative which calms inflammations of the skin. This had the effect of soothing the itching but brought about little change in the actual spots.

The poor woman was literally in despair at the failure of all her efforts, every new treatment having proved yet another disappointment, yet another setback. And no wonder: her face was swollen, purple, criss-crossed with a tight network of red capillary vessels and covered with spots a millimetre in diameter from her hairline down to her neck.

So far as I could judge the skin was also atrophic, as happens when too great a quantity of corticosteroids is applied over too long a period; this should always be avoided in the case of rosacea, firstly because it does very little good, secondly because it damages the skin, and lastly because it could even cause outbreaks of spots similar to rosacea, thereby adding insult to injury!

Her rosacea was therefore unusually acute, both in extent and in its resistance to normally effective treatment which she had followed to the letter.

I asked her to get her teeth X-rayed, hoping against hope that this would disclose some abscesses. To be honest, I don't know what I would have done had there not been any. There were two, both of them enormous. They were treated without delay, and six weeks later she was completely cured and overcome with joy and relief. So was I!

Not many cases are so dramatic and difficult to treat, thank goodness. Often when a patient has obviously become allergic to some microbe, the most meticulous search fails to disclose its focus: since it isn't causing an infection, it's impossible to find. Here, the so-called 'wide-spectrum' antibiotics act as miracle drugs. Attacking as they do almost all microbes wherever they are found, one can be almost sure of hitting the right one. With the use of Tetracyclines, the spots clear up completely in eight days.

Unfortunately this remarkable improvement seldom lasts; the outbreaks of spots tend to recur within a week to a month after the completion of the treatment. There is only one way to prevent such relapses: to keep the antibiotics going and sustain the cure by means of long-term treatment in very weak doses. The idea of this provokes much the same objections as in acne patients:

'You're surely not suggesting that I go on taking antibiotics for the rest of my life! I'll build up a resistance to them and then, if I ever need them for anything else, they won't have any effect.'

I've already exploded this myth; there's no point in repeating myself. What is true for the acne sufferer is equally true for rosacea; all the more so, in fact, since the dosage needed to keep rosacea at bay is even weaker: one capsule morning and night, one or two days a week — a weekly total which is half or one third the dose that you would absorb daily if you were taking the same antibiotic for an infection. It's such an insignificant amount that you won't notice it, and it has the added advantage of keeping your skin in excellent condition.

One of the nurses at my clinic in Paris was a patient of mine for twenty years; she suffered from very bad rosacea which had started when she was twenty-seven years old. She had responded well to five short eight-day courses of antibiotics spread over three months and remained quite free from the complaint for the next four years, which goes to show that antibiotics can give prolonged protection. Then she fell ill with pleurisy and, at the same time, her rosacea reappeared. Without consulting me, she tried a series of other treatments, all to no avail, including some twenty applications of carbon dioxide snow and six sessions of radiotherapy on the nape of the neck designed to act on the sympathetic nervous system. She finally returned to see me after more than two years of repeated failures. As soon as she was back on antibiotics, all was well again.

Two resorcin exfoliations performed at two weeks' interval had had an excellent effect on her facial redness and meant that I could quickly reduce the antibiotics to the minimum effective dose. In her case this consisted of six capsules a week, and she couldn't do without it: as soon as she stopped the treatment — and she made

the experiment voluntarily two or three times – the spots returned.
Fifteen years of Tetracycline at this low dosage convinced her that
the treatment was quite safe; taking it became second nature to her,
and she no longer had the slightest wish to stop it.

I should add that exactly the same results are obtained in men
with an equal rate of success, that is, 90 per cent; this is quite un-
related to what happens in acne, where the same antibiotics only
show an improvement in one case in ten.

I should also explain what I mean by improvement: in the case
of rosacea you can expect the outbreaks of spots to stop completely,
whereas in the case of acne the spots will become smaller, fewer
and less frequent, but will not completely disappear.

I have kept until last two particularly unsightly diseases, both
related to rosacea in so far as the causes and the mechanism determining them are concerned, but both presenting very different
symptoms.

One is peculiar to women and never occurs in men; conversely,
the other is peculiar to men and never occurs in women.

ACNE OF THE CHIN

The first is known as *deep nodular acne of the chin in the adult female*,
which would be an accurate description were it not for the fact
that, as with rosacea, it's not an acne at all, but an allergy caused
by microbes.

It's a particularly infuriating complaint: the large red spots –
hard, deep-seated and painful – only occur two or three at a time
and at irregular intervals; but, once formed, they last for a couple
of weeks, or even a month, so that the unfortunate sufferer knows
no respite between one outbreak and the next.

It has been observed that the rhythm of the outbreaks often
follows that of ovulation or the monthly periods; but you can't
even count on this, and you may be sure that when there's an important social occasion and you want to look your best, you'll wake
up to find that one of these insufferable lumps has treacherously
appeared during the night. While they usually clear up without
discharging pus, they can leave very nasty scars, especially if you
pick at them or squeeze them.

Treatment is exactly the same as for rosacea.

RHINOPHYMA

The second of these complaints goes by the barbarous name of rhinophyma; in fact, it's a disfiguring form of rosacea of the nose: the skin becomes thick, lumpy, deep red and covered in spots and widely dilated capillaries. The nose can swell to enormous size, becoming turgescent and purple-veined, especially around the nostrils. The slightest nick bleeds profusely. Rhinophyma may be associated with rosacea of the rest of the face or remain isolated in the middle of an otherwise clear complexion.

This excrescence is a real burden to sufferers, not only because of its hideousness but also because of its associations: a man with a red nose is automatically assumed to be a man who likes the bottle. Far from being synonymous with drunkenness, rhinophyma often attacks the soberest of men; indeed, sufferers tend to drink less than most people, since the least drop of alcohol is enough to light up the beacon they carry in the middle of their faces.

Antibiotics are not of much help in this case; one must have recourse to surgery: the surface of the nose is literally shaved off with a razor. The operation is always performed under anaesthetic; it is delicate and bleeding is profuse.

The epidermis is either left to repair itself, in which case there is scar-tissue, or else a fine skin-graft is taken from the thigh. These days many cosmetic surgeons prefer the latter method because it has the advantage of covering the nose with healthy skin; but it has a somewhat patchwork effect because the skin-graft has a different texture from the surrounding skin.

Nevertheless, thanks to one or other of these methods, the nose can be brought back to normal size and colour, and this, for anyone who has had rhinophyma, amounts to a veritable resurrection.

DISORDERS OF THE HYPODERMIS

The fatty tissue represents 14 per cent of the body-weight in men between the ages of twenty-five and thirty, and 32 per cent in women of similar age, or a mean of 20 per cent (see Table III).

TABLE III   *Distribution of separate constituent elements*
of the body according to corpulence

	Normal subject %	Thin subject %	Fat subject %
Fats	20	2	50
Intra-cellular water	43	49	25
Extra-cellular water	15	23	12
Intra-cellular solids	16	20	7
Minerals	6	6	6

Table after Professor Justin-Besançon.

In both sexes, two-thirds of the fatty tissue is found in the deepest layer of the skin, the hypodermis, and this is the reason why a normal woman is always rounder in shape and better-covered than a normal man.

Seen under a microscope, hypodermic tissue resembles a sponge: dividing the spherical cavities are *septa*, or the connective tissue lining, in which the numerous blood-vessels and fine nerve-fibres travel; each cavity contains a fat cell or 'lipocyte' packed with tiny globules of fat.

As we have seen in the first part of this book (but it does no harm to remind ourselves of it), the fatty hypodermis acts as built-in protection, like a well-sprung mattress, for the underlying tissues: the muscles, tendons and bones; it insulates the internal environment from external variations in temperature; it constitutes a reserve of food upon which the organism can draw as and when it needs – in the case of starvation, for example, or when a task requires an additional supply of 'combustible fuel' in order to compensate for lost energy.

In addition, it constitutes a reserve of water, of which, depending on the part of the body, the fatty tissue retains between 12 and 30 per cent; this important reservoir acts as a regulator for the total fluid circulating in the blood and lymph and between the cells.

The hypodermis is subject to a number of different disorders, only three of which concern us here:
— anomalies in the amount of fat contained in the hypodermis: an excess in the case of *obesity*, a deficiency in the case of *leanness*;

— anomalies in the hydration of the hypodermis: the characteristics of the condition known as 'cellulite'.

OBESITY AND EXCESSIVE LEANNESS

Normality, from the point of view of weight, is the result of the food-intake being precisely adapted to the needs of the organism.

To a doctor, therefore, obesity and leanness represent an imbalance between intake and output. In obesity, the intake exceeds the output and the organism is hoarding food; in leanness, the organism is squandering food and the output exceeds the intake.

This imbalance creates a disproportion between a person's weight and his or her height. This can be calculated mathematically in relation to what we call *ideal weight* and *standard weight*.

Ideal weight is that which, in a person of given age, height and sex, allows for the fullest possible physical and intellectual activity, offers the maximum life expectancy, ensures well-being and makes for a well-proportioned figure.

It is arrived at by formulae whose value lies not in enabling one to recognise obesity or leanness—these can be seen at a glance—but in helping one to assess the degree to which people are overweight or underweight and, with patients under treatment, to keep track of their progress.

Lorentz has proposed the simplest formula:

$$\text{Ideal weight} = H - 100 - \frac{(H - 150)}{4}$$

where H is the height in centimetres.

If you apply this formula to a man 1·76 metres tall, you get:

$$176 - 100 - \frac{(176 - 150)}{4} = 69·5 \text{ kilograms}$$

The values given for ideal weight in this formula are less valid in the case of women: indeed, by the same calculation, a woman 1·70 metres tall should weigh 65 kilograms; without being obese, a woman of this weight would definitely be on the plump side for her height. The reason is that Lorentz's formula doesn't take into account the weight of the body-frame. Another formula has been suggested, taking the circumference of the wrist (C) to represent the body-frame as a whole:

$$\text{Ideal weight} = \frac{H - 100 + 4C}{2}$$

According to this formula, the ideal weight for a woman 1·70 metres tall, with a wrist measurement of 13 centimetres, is 61 kilograms, which is both more realistic and closer to present-day aesthetic standards.

There are tables which show the ideal weight considered to give maximum life-expectancy, taking into account the height and type of body-frame of men and women aged twenty-five and over. One such table was published in 1959 by a group of life insurance companies in America. (Reproduced as Table IV.)

Standard weight is calculated from statistics based on the study of a large group of people considered to be normal in weight. A glance at Table V will show that the standard average weight of a woman 1·70 metres tall ranges from 61·6 kilograms between the ages of twenty-five and twenty-nine to 68·4 kilograms between the ages of forty and forty-nine. For a small-framed woman of similar age, however, the ideal weight would not exceed 57·5 kilograms.

Such variations show that these figures should not be taken too literally. They are orders of magnitude, for the purposes of assessment and comparison, nothing more.

Nevertheless, taking both standard and ideal weights for an adult of given height aged between twenty and thirty as a reference, to be 10 per cent over this is to show the first signs of obesity; if you exceed it by 20 per cent, you are frankly obese. Conversely, you are on the thin side if your actual weight is 10 per cent less than your ideal weight.

The complex problems associated with being seriously overweight or underweight are well outside the scope of this book, and I don't intend to go into them here.

Certain significant points are worth mentioning, however, because although obesity and leanness appear to be opposites, their causes, contrary to what one might think at first sight, are not.

Both conditions amount to a disfigurement, the more so, obviously, the more pronounced they are: a very thin person is no more attractive to look at than a very fat one.

But while obesity is a disease, excessive leanness is not: it is a physical state. In fact, with the exception of those cases where the loss of weight is due to a serious internal disease, whether organic

TABLE IV *Ideal adult weight*

Height (in cm with shoes)	Ideal weight (in kg, dressed) 25 and over MEN			Height (in cm with shoes)	Ideal weight (in kg, dressed) 25 and over WOMEN		
	Light frame	Medium frame	Heavy frame		Light frame	Medium frame	Heavy frame
157	50·5-54·2	53·3-58·2	56·9-63·7	148	42·0-44·8	43·8-48·9	47·4-54·3
158	51·1-54·7	53·8-58·9	57·4-64·2	149	42·3-45·4	44·1-49·4	47·8-54·9
159	51·6-55·2	54·3-59·6	58·0-64·8	150	42·7-45·9	44·5-50·0	48·2-55·4
160	52·2-55·8	54·9-60·3	58·5-65·3	151	43·0-46·4	45·1-50·5	48·7-55·9
161	52·7-56·3	55·4-60·9	59·0-66·0	152	43·4-47·0	45·6-51·0	49·2-56·5
162	53·2-56·9	55·9-61·4	59·6-66·7	153	43·9-47·5	46·1-51·6	49·8-57·0
163	53·8-57·4	56·5-61·9	60·1-67·5	154	44·4-48·0	46·7-52·1	50·3-57·6
164	54·3-57·9	57·0-62·5	60·7-68·2	155	44·9-48·6	47·2-52·6	50·8-58·1
165	54·9-58·5	57·6-63·0	61·2-68·9	156	45·4-49·1	47·7-53·2	51·3-58·6
166	55·4-59·2	58·1-63·7	61·7-69·6	157	46·0-49·6	48·2-53·7	51·9-59·1
167	55·9-59·9	58·6-64·4	62·3-70·3	158	46·5-50·2	48·8-54·3	52·4-59·7
168	56·5-60·6	59·2-65·1	62·9-71·1	159	47·1-50·7	49·3-54·8	53·0-60·2
169	57·2-61·3	59·9-65·8	63·6-72·0	160	47·6-51·2	49·9-55·3	53·5-60·8
170	57·9-62·0	60·7-66·6	64·3-72·9	161	48·2-51·8	50·4-56·0	54·0-61·5
171	58·6-62·7	61·4-67·4	65·1-73·8	162	48·7-52·3	51·0-56·8	54·6-62·2
172	59·4-63·4	62·1-68·3	66·0-74·7	163	49·2-52·9	51·5-57·5	55·2-62·9
173	60·1-64·2	62·8-69·1	66·9-75·5	164	49·8-53·4	52·0-58·2	55·9-63·7
174	60·8-64·9	63·5-69·9	67·6-76·2	165	50·3-53·9	52·6-58·9	56·7-64·4
175	61·5-65·6	64·2-70·6	68·3-76·9	166	50·8-54·6	53·3-59·8	57·3-65·1
176	62·2-66·4	64·9-71·3	69·0-77·6	167	51·4-55·3	54·0-60·7	58·1-65·8
177	62·9-67·3	65·7-72·0	69·7-78·4	168	52·0-56·0	54·7-61·5	58·8-66·5
178	63·6-68·2	66·4-72·8	70·4-79·1	169	52·7-56·8	55·4-62·2	59·5-67·2
179	64·4-68·9	67·1-73·6	71·2-80·0	170	53·4-57·5	56·1-62·9	60·2-68·6
180	65·1-69·6	67·8-74·5	71·9-80·9	171	54·1-58·2	56·8-63·6	60·9-68·6
181	65·8-70·3	68·5-75·4	72·7-81·8	172	54·8-58·9	57·5-64·3	61·6-69·3
182	66·5-71·0	69·2-76·3	73·6-82·7	173	55·5-59·6	58·3-65·1	62·3-70·1
183	67·2-71·8	69·9-77·2	74·5-83·6	174	56·3-60·3	59·0-65·8	63·1-70·8
184	67·9-72·5	70·7-78·1	75·2-84·5	175	57·0-61·0	59·7-66·5	63·8-71·5
185	68·6-73·2	71·4-79·0	75·9-85·4	176	57·7-61·9	60·4-67·2	64·5-72·3
186	69·4-74·0	72·1-79·9	76·7-86·2	177	58·4-62·8	61·1-67·8	65·2-73·2
187	70·1-74·9	72·8-80·8	77·6-87·1	178	59·1-63·6	61·8-68·6	65·9-74·1
188	70·8-75·8	73·5-81·7	78·5-88·0	179	59·8-64·4	62·5-69·3	66·6-75·0
189	71·5-76·5	74·4-82·6	79·4-88·9	180	60·5-65·1	63·3-70·1	67·3-75·9
190	72·2-77·2	75·3-83·5	80·3-89·8	181	61·3-65·8	64·0-70·8	68·1-76·8
191	72·9-77·9	76·2-84·4	81·1-90·7	182	62·0-66·5	64·7-71·5	68·8-77·7
192	73·6-78·6	77·1-85·3	81·8-91·6	183	62·7-67·2	65·4-72·2	69·5-78·6
193	74·4-79·3	78·0-86·1	82·5-92·5	184	63·4-67·9	66·1-72·9	70·2-79·5
194	75·1-80·1	78·9-87·0	83·2-93·4	185	64·1-68·6	66·8-73·6	70·9-80·4
195	75·8-80·8	79·8-87·9	84·0-94·3				

NOTE: 1 inch = 2·54 cm; 1 kg = 2·2 lbs.

TABLE V   *Standard mean adult weight*

Height (in cm with shoes)	Average weight (in kg, dressed) MEN							
	15-16 years	17-19 years	20-24 years	25-29 years	30-39 years	40-49 years	50-59 years	60-69 years
153	44·9	51·7	55·7	58·4	59·7	61·1	62·0	60·7
154	45·6	52·1	56·2	58·9	60·3	61·6	62·5	61·2
155	46·3	52·6	56·7	59·5	60·8	62·2	63·1	61·7
156	47·2	53·2	57·2	60·0	61·3	62·7	63·6	62·2
157	48·1	53·7	57·8	60·5	61·9	63·2	64·1	62·8
158	49·0	54·3	58·4	61·2	62·5	63·9	64·7	63·3
159	49·9	55·1	59·1	61·9	63·2	64·6	65·2	63·9
160	50·8	55·8	59·9	62·6	63·9	65·3	65·8	64·4
161	51·7	56·5	60·6	63·1	64·7	66·0	66·5	65·1
162	52·6	57·2	61·3	63·7	65·4	66·7	67·2	65·8
163	53·5	58·0	61·9	64·2	66·1	67·5	67·9	66·6
164	54·4	58·7	62·5	64·8	66·8	68·2	68·6	67·3
165	55·3	59·4	63·0	65·3	67·5	68·9	69·4	68·0
166	56·1	60·1	63·5	66·0	68·2	69·6	70·0	68·7
167	57·0	60·8	64·1	66·7	68·9	70·3	70·8	69·4
168	57·9	61·6	64·6	67·3	69·7	71·1	71·5	70·2
169	58·8	62·2	65·1	67·9	70·4	72·0	72·4	71·1
170	59·7	62·9	65·7	68·4	71·1	72·9	73·3	72·0
171	60·6	63·6	66·4	69·1	71·8	73·6	74·1	72·7
172	61·5	64·3	67·1	69·8	72·5	74·3	74·8	73·4
173	62·4	65·1	67·8	70·5	73·2	75·0	75·5	74·2
174	63·3	65·8	68·5	71·2	73·9	75·8	76·2	75·1
175	64·2	66·5	69·2	71·9	74·7	76·5	76·9	76·0
176	64·9	67·2	69·9	72·6	75·5	77·3	77·8	76·9
177	65·7	67·9	70·6	73·4	76·4	78·2	78·7	77·8
178	66·4	68·6	71·4	74·1	77·3	79·1	79·6	78·7
179	67·1	69·3	72·1	74·8	78·0	79·8	80·5	79·5
180	67·8	70·1	72·8	75·5	78·7	80·5	81·3	80·4
181	68·5	70·9	73·6	76·3	79·5	81·3	82·2	81·3
182	69·2	71·8	74·5	77·2	80·4	82·2	83·1	82·2
183	70·0	72·7	75·4	78·1	81·3	83·1	84·0	83·1
184	70·9	73·4	76·1	79·0	82·0	83·8	84·7	84·0
185	71·7	74·1	76·8	79·9	82·7	84·5	85·4	84·9
186	72·6	74·8	77·5	80·8	83·5	85·3	86·2	85·8
187	73·5	75·5	78·2	81·7	84·4	86·2	87·1	86·7
188	74·4	76·2	79·0	82·6	85·3	87·1	88·0	87·6
189	75·3	76·9	79·7	83·3	86·2	88·0	88·9	88·5
190	76·2	77·7	80·4	84·0	87·1	88·9	89·8	89·4
191	77·1	78·4	81·0	84·7	88·1	89·9	90·8	90·3
192	78·0	79·1	81·5	85·4	89·2	91·0	91·9	91·4
193	—	79·8	82·1	86·2	90·2	92·0	92·9	92·5
194	—	80·5	82·6	86·9	91·3	93·1	94·0	93·6
195	—	81·2	83·2	87·6	92·4	94·2	95·1	94·6

TABLE V *Standard mean adult weight*

Height (in cm with shoes)	*Average weight (in kg, dressed)* WOMEN							
	15-16 years	17-19 years	20-24 years	25-29 years	30-39 years	40-49 years	50-59 years	60-69 years
148	44·4	45·3	46·6	48·9	52·4	55·6	56·9	57·8
149	44·9	45·8	47·2	49·4	52·8	55·9	57·3	58·2
150	45·4	46·3	47·7	50·0	53·1	56·3	57·7	58·6
151	46·0	46·9	48·2	50·5	53·7	56·9	58·2	58·9
152	46·5	47·4	48·8	51·0	54·2	57·4	58·8	59·3
153	47·1	48·1	49·4	51·6	54·8	57·9	59·3	59·8
154	47·9	48·8	50·1	52·1	55·3	58·5	59·8	60·3
155	48·6	49·5	50·8	52·6	55·8	59·0	60·4	60·8
156	49·3	50·2	51·3	53·2	56·3	59·5	60·9	61·3
157	50·0	50·9	51·9	53·7	56·9	60·0	61·4	61·9
158	50·6	51·5	52·4	54·3	57·4	60·6	62·1	62·5
159	51·1	52·1	53·0	54·8	58·0	61·1	62·8	63·2
160	51·7	52·6	53·5	55·3	58·5	61·7	63·5	63·9
161	52·2	53·3	54·0	55·9	59·0	62·4	64·2	64·7
162	52·8	54·0	54·6	56·5	59·6	63·1	64·9	65·4
163	53·4	54·8	55·2	57·0	60·1	63·8	65·7	66·1
164	54·1	55·5	55·9	57·7	60·7	64·3	66·4	66·8
165	54·8	56·2	56·6	58·5	61·2	64·8	67·1	67·5
166	55·5	56·7	57·3	59·2	61·9	65·5	67·8	68·2
167	56·2	57·3	58·1	59·9	62·6	66·2	68·5	68·9
168	56·9	57·8	58·7	60·5	63·2	66·9	69·2	69·7
169	57·4	58·3	59·2	61·1	63·8	67·6	69·9	70·4
170	58·0	58·9	59·8	61·6	64·3	68·4	70·6	71·1
171	58·6	59·6	60·5	62·3	65·0	69·1	71·3	71·8
172	59·4	60·3	61·2	63·0	65·7	69·8	72·1	72·5
173	60·1	61·0	61·9	63·7	66·4	70·5	72·8	73·2
174	60·8	61·7	62·6	64·4	67·1	71·2	73·5	73·9
175	61·5	62·4	63·3	65·1	67·9	71·9	74·2	74·7
176	62·2	63·1	64·0	65·8	68·6	72·8	75·1	75·4
177	62·9	63·8	64·7	66·6	69·3	73·7	75·9	76·1
178	63·6	64·6	65·5	67·3	70·0	74·6	76·8	76·8
179	—	65·5	66·4	68·2	70·9	75·5	77·7	—
180	—	66·4	67·3	69·1	71·8	76·4	78·6	—
181	—	67·3	68·2	70·0	72·7	77·2	79·6	—
182	—	68·2	69·1	70·9	73·6	78·1	80·7	—
183	—	69·1	70·0	71·8	74·5	79·0	81·8	—
184	—	70·0	70·9	72·7	75·4	79·9	82·9	—
185	—	70·9	71·8	73·6	76·3	80·8	83·9	—

or psychological—when it is more correct to talk of wasting—the thin person is extremely healthy.

On the other hand, the encroachment of fat makes a person who is seriously overweight vulnerable to a mass of complications affecting the kidneys, liver and circulation of the blood, including high blood-pressure. According to the statistics produced by the Metropolitan Life Insurance Company, the frequency of heart-attacks is 40 per cent higher in obese people than in those of normal weight.

HEREDITARY LEANNESS

While the fat person is short of breath, inactive, easily tired and quick to fall ill, the thin person is active, dynamic, very resistant to fatigue physically and sexually, blessed with a good appetite, rarely ill, and lives to a ripe old age. Thin women are no less energetic and tough than lean men. But while the lean man is usually perfectly content to be so, the lean woman is constantly dissatisfied with her skinny ribs and thighs, her 'salt-cellars' and her underdeveloped breasts.

As constitutionally thin men and women don't suffer from glandular or similar disorders, there is little hope of their gaining weight. *Their leanness is part of their inheritance*, and whenever one yields to the insistence of patients who are worried by it and attempts to treat them, one is only building up false hopes: should a patient succeed, at the cost of painstaking and extremely prolonged efforts, in gaining a few kilograms, the extra weight will be lost again in half the time taken to put it on; and more often than not, both patient and doctor will have lost interest long before the smallest gain has been achieved.

OBESITY, THE DISEASE OF SURFEIT

Again, in the case of obesity it is a different matter: although the excess fat may sometimes be constitutional in origin, *its essential cause is always linked to food*; not only in the quantity of food taken in, but also in its quality and the way in which it is absorbed.

It follows from this now universally accepted fact that all fat people can lose weight with the help of the appropriate diet, provided that they adhere to it.

One cannot be too wary of bogus or imitation diets—no diet

which has not been prescribed by a doctor can do any good – and of so-called 'shock' diets.

The number of times I've heard:

'I don't eat bread, I never drink with meals, yet I never seem to be able to lose any weight.' It's not surprising: measures like these are hopelessly inadequate. Patients sometimes ask my advice on how to lose weight, and, even though the question is rather outside my province, before referring them to a specialist, I first go over their problems with them.

The typical woman patient will always begin by declaring that she doesn't eat a thing. I gently point out that she looks rather too well for someone who eats nothing at all; if she fasted completely she would look like a Nazi concentration camp survivor. There weren't any cases of obesity in Buchenwald or Dachau! I then get her to itemise her 'starvation' diet, in order to make her realise that what she calls 'nothing' amounts to 2500 calories a day.

One such patient had cut out all starch, but was eating 2 kilograms of fruit a day: apples, pears, peaches, bananas, nectarines, cherries, apricots, strawberries, according to season. For every 100 grams of fruit she was eating 15 grams of sugar; this amounted to a daily intake of 300 grams of sugar, or 1200 calories,* not counting her half-litre of wine at 375 calories, the oil in her salad dressing at 100 calories, grilled steaks at 400 calories, etc.

REDUCING THE INTAKE

It wasn't surprising that she hadn't managed to lose any weight when you consider that the calorie-intake must be reduced to between 1000 and 1200 calories a day to have any effect.

A slimming diet cannot be improvised; only specialists in nutritional problems are qualified to say what form it should take. A person's diet should take into account the seriousness of the disorder to be treated, as well as his or her age and way of life; it must also be properly balanced in order to avoid the problems which can easily arise if an indispensable element of diet is too drastically reduced. Care must be taken to see that weight-loss is not achieved at the cost of muscle-wastage, by making sure that the

---

* In physics, a calorie is the unit of measurement of heat given off by combustion; that is, the energy provided by the body; the normal requirement for a healthy adult weighing 65 kilograms is 2500 calories a day. (A-B)

supply of protein doesn't fall below 1 gram for every kilogram of ideal weight — the equivalent of eating about 200 grams of meat a day (protein is one of the constituent elements of living matter: eggs, meat, fish and milk are the chief sources of protein in our food); nor should the sugar intake be allowed to drop below 50 grams a day, or you risk poor absorption of protein; and so on.

Contrary to popular belief, you can drink as much water as you like — whether between meals or not is immaterial. There is only one exception to this otherwise total freedom, and that is in the case of so-called 'spongy' obesity, caused by water-retention, where the patient swells when active and deflates when resting, a condition wholly confined to women. When the total amount of liquid absorbed daily (including coffee, tea and soup) is measured and compared with the amount of urine excreted over a period of six days during which the intake of all non-measurable water, such as that contained in fruit, is prohibited, the results show that consumption and excretion balance out as long as a certain volume of liquid in every twenty-four hours is not exceeded: usually between 500–600 grams. Above this amount the balance-sheet is in deficit, the patient excreting noticeably less than she has drunk. By reducing the fluid intake of such patients over a given period, and at the same time cutting down their salt to make the restriction easier, significant and long-lasting improvements can be obtained.

Otherwise there is no need to prevent patients from drinking all the water, milkless tea or black coffee they want, especially as the desire for water diminishes as the number of calories is reduced: it has been established that our fluid absorption is roughly equal to that of our calorie absorption. On the other hand, it should not be forgotten that a litre of beer contains 450 calories and a litre of 10° proof wine, 750 calories.

INCREASING THE OUTPUT

But one cannot slim merely by reducing the intake of food; you must also increase the output of energy. Except in the case of water-retention, where, paradoxically, exercise actually promotes a gain in weight, regular, sensible physical exercise is essential.

Some people claim that physical exercise only awakens and stimulates the appetite. It is sometimes said that you need to walk for thirty-six hours or spend seven hours sawing wood in order to lose 100 grams of fat! This is a fallacy; you don't see many corpulent lumberjacks or navvies; corpulence is rare in people who do physical labour. The people who are overweight are those in sedentary occupations.

A normal person uses up between 1·5 and 2·5 calories a minute doing light work, and 12·5 calories or more doing heavy work; thus a man who sits at a desk reading or writing is using up 1·5 calories a minute, whereas a man who is rowing or swimming is using up 15 or 20. By the same token, everyday activities such as getting up, dressing, and preparing for bed account for between 2·5 and 4 calories a minute.

Since people who are overweight use up on average 15 per cent more calories than people of normal weight for the same activities, it is a simple matter for them to burn up 300–500 extra calories a day. But they must be careful how they set about it, for they need to avoid putting too much strain on their heart and arteries.

From every point of view, the best possible exercise is walking over flat ground: not only can speed and distance be regulated, but it is suitable for all ages. Furthermore, it is always possible to find the time and opportunity, whereas we all know that physical jerks in the bedroom are rarely kept up for long.

Massage does little good, unless it is to help tone up wasted muscles or make stiff joints supple.

As for sweating, either in a sauna or a Turkish bath, the loss of water is rapidly nullified by a massive consumption of beverages by way of compensation.

Cold baths are much more advisable: they withdraw a certain amount of heat, and hence calories, from the body; and when they can be taken in a swimming-pool, they combine the benefits of physical exercise with those of the cooling process.

RE-LEARNING HOW TO EAT

People who are overweight often ask to be given 'appetite suppressors', diuretics or thyroid extracts to supplement their dieting.

'Appetite suppressors' are, technically speaking, anti-hunger agents which stimulate the central nervous system. They often cause dizziness and insomnia, and, in my opinion, contribute more to the failure of a treatment than to its success: the treatment of obesity doesn't consist only of bringing about a loss of weight through a restricted diet, *it is also and above all a question of re-education in eating habits.* The patient must be weaned away from and cured of his or her obsession with food; he or she must re-learn how to eat in order to live, instead of living in order to eat. Without the will-power to do this, any improvement is bound to be short-lived. Now, appetite suppressors are a substitute for will-power: we leave up to them the effort we have neither the courage nor the real desire to make for ourselves. We abdicate. That is why, even if obliged to use them to get the cure off to a good start, one should never allow a patient to persist with them for long.

Nor is there any valid reason for using diuretics unless they are justified by cardiac or renal disorders. They cause a copious excretion of urine which is immediately counter-balanced by water-retention. There is no point in taking a step forward only to take the same step back again immediately afterwards.

As for thyroid extracts, they are positively dangerous when, as is usually the case, the thyroid gland is functioning normally. *Except in rare cases, obesity is not a disease which is glandular in origin.*

Generally speaking, therefore, one can say that all these drugs, contra-indicated for a number of different reasons and not without risk, positively hinder the patient from following his or her diet properly.

The success of any cure for overweight depends wholly on the strict observance of the prescribed diet, and the most difficult thing of all is to make people understand this and carry it out.

'CELLULITE'

In 1973 I was watching a television programme on the treatment of 'cellulite' in which someone remarked that 'the almost obsessional fear that women have of cellulite began with the fashion for wearing trousers, or rather, trousers cut like men's.'

I didn't altogether agree. The horror of 'cellulite' dates back to a period long before trousers became fashionable for women. In the days when skirts were down to the ankles women still sought the help of doctors and masseuses: when the time came for the skirt to be removed, dimpled, bulging thighs were hardly likely to excite the admiration of husband or lover, or even fellow bathers on the beach. True, the advent of tight-fitting trousers – like those blue-jeans worn in the bath and dried on the body until moulded to it – was an added inducement.

But we should also recognise that with 'cellulite', as with other unaesthetic conditions, not only fashion but the desire for perfection, and the repugnance shown towards disease, disfigurement and infirmity in our consumer society play a not inconsiderable part in the search for treatment. We are demanding more and more of medicine. We expect it to solve all our problems, 'cellulite' included.

Unfortunately, there's a hitch: even when we know how and why a particular condition comes about, we don't always have the means to correct it. And when, as is the case with 'cellulite', we don't know how and why it develops, we must be honest and admit that its treatment – really effective treatment, that is – has still to be discovered. The proof is that we don't know how to prevent it.

For the present, therefore, we have to be content with more or less empirical methods whose results are unreliable, sometimes partial, always short-lived.

Even though men are not immune from it, 'cellulite' is essentially a feminine affliction.

'Cellulite' should be distinguished from obesity. The two phenomena may co-exist, and indeed always do co-exist in the case of certain obese conditions where the fat, limited to the lower half of the body, caricatures the distinctive female contours of hips and thighs.

But 'cellulite' can exist without any sign of obesity: it can occur on the neck, arms, thoracic cage, breasts, thighs, inside of the knees and lower third of the legs. It is when concentrated around the hips and the outside of the thighs, rather like a pair of jodhpurs, that it's most troublesome to women who want to wear trousers.

'Cellulitic' skin has a quilted appearance which is accentuated by the contraction of the muscles or by pinching. The latter is usually painful, and some women even complain of spontaneous sensitivity to a greater or lesser degree. It is embarrassment as much as anything else which sends them to the doctor.

We know very little about the nature of 'cellulite' other than that it constitutes a chronic alteration of the cellulo-fatty tissue of the hypodermis, but without any accompanying inflammation.

L

HOW 'CELLULITE' STARTS

'Cellulite' appears to develop in three stages:

1 First, fluids from the blood and lymph infiltrate the septa between the fat 'lobules'. At the same time the fat cells in these lobules become charged with fat.

2 Next, the cells become water-logged and the fibrous tissue proliferates; the walls of the blood-vessels themselves swell with water, causing their dimensions to shrink and the circulation of the blood to slow down. In this rather distended, water-logged tissue, very special substances belonging to the chemical family of polymers (as do plastics and nylon), condense and form a sort of gel which coats the connective fibres.

3 Lastly, the hardening (or 'induration' as it is called) of the hypodermis reaches its maximum: 'sclerosis' has set in: the thickened fibrous mat forms wide interwoven bands adhering at their base to the muscle sheaths and at their top to the dermis, while the much-swollen fat cells tend to bulge outwards from the spaces in the fibrous network.

The skin's quilted appearance, like orange-peel, accentuated whenever the muscles contract, is the result of this combination of cellular swelling and sclerosis of the connective fibres.

WHAT CAUSES 'CELLULITE'

We can only guess at the causes of this type of skin damage.

Circulation trouble in the veins of the legs has been blamed; but this often exists quite independently of 'cellulite' and doesn't imply a relationship of cause and effect between these two disorders.

Some people believe that it could be due to stasis, that is a slowing-down of the circulation of the blood in the tiny arterial capillaries which may be encouraged by posture defects such as flat feet or the hollowing of the back through a tilting of the pelvis combined with insufficient muscle-tone in the buttocks.

It is probable that the hormones play a part, especially the female hormone, because it is a contributory cause of water-retention and congestive phenomena; but this has yet to be proved.

What is certain, on the other hand, is that the mechanism leading to obesity is not the same as that leading to 'cellulite', because treatments effective in the former are completely useless in the latter.

And while one can combat obesity by treating its cause, one cannot do so in the case of 'cellulite' because the exact cause is a mystery, hence the extremely dubious efficacy of the numerous treatments which have been devised and whose very multiplicity is suspect.

Sometimes a patient is advised to combine a general treatment with local treatment, sometimes to restrict treatment to local applications.

THE PROS AND CONS OF INTERNAL TREATMENTS

Some practitioners believe in internal treatment; they advise dieting (which is valueless since 'cellulite' is almost never associated with obesity), vitamins, hormones, appetite suppressors and diuretics.

I've no objection to vitamins; they may not do any good, but at least they do no harm.

Hormones are far less innocent; oestrogens even have the reputation of aggravating certain conditions and people are quick to blame contraceptive pills containing oestrogen for causing this unpleasant effect. In fact, I know of hundreds of women who have used these drugs for years without suffering any such ill-effects. And in the case of those women with 'cellulite' who suffer from water-retention before their periods, accompanied by swelling of the breasts and stomach due to an over-secretion of oestrogen by the ovaries, the removal of these symptoms by the appropriate treatment doesn't entail a corresponding cure of the 'cellulite', which would be the case were there a connection between high oestrogens and 'cellulite'.

The thyroid hormone (thyroxine), when taken by mouth, is no more effective in 'cellulite' than it is in obesity and entails the same undesirable side-effects of palpitations, diarrhoea, nervous tension, insomnia and unhealthy loss of weight.

Cortisone derivatives (corticosteroids) are positively dangerous and should not be used unless absolutely necessary, which is not the case here.

Lastly, the remarks I made about the use of diuretics and appetite suppressors in obesity apply equally to 'cellulite'; I shall not go over them again. But I must emphasise that great care is needed in the use of these drugs should one venture to try them.

EXTERNAL TREATMENT

To sum up, all that can be done for 'cellulite', at present, is to treat it purely locally.

And as there is no one medicament which gives positive and unarguable results, several are combined at once in the hope of increasing the chances of success. Some of these 'cocktails' contain as many as seven different products. None of them can work miracles.

The most popular is a mixture of a mild diuretic, for getting rid of the water; an enzyme, for dissolving the gel which coats the connective fibres, and a hormone, thyroxine, intended to metabolise the fats of the cellulitic mass. The thyroid hormone, thyroxine, when applied locally and within the prescribed limits, does not have the same side-effects as when taken internally.

TREATMENT BY INJECTION

Injections may be made by means of a long needle inserted progressively beneath the skin parallel to the surface, depositing its contents as it goes. These so-called 'creeping' injections are rather painful and it is advisable to add a local anaesthetic to the combination of medicaments.

They can also be done with a special device, comprising a hollow plate to which are attached eighteen fine needles between 4–8 millimetres long. The fluid to be injected is thus introduced into the hypodermis at eighteen separate points simultaneously and disperses uniformly. It's an ingenious system, allowing a given surface to be treated at one time and avoiding the unpleasant sensation of the probing needle in the 'creeping' type of injection.

TREATMENT BY IONTOPHORESIS

Special electrical apparatus can be used to introduce medicaments in solution into the skin by means of a current passing between two plates. This method is known as iontophoresis. It also ensures an even distribution of the medicaments, and furthermore is quite painless.

Either method, injection or iontophoresis, usually requires two sessions a week over eight to ten weeks: for a woman with a job, it's a time-consuming business.

TREATMENT BY FRICTION

For those women without the time to spare, there is a form of treatment that can be undertaken at home, under a doctor's supervision. Having warmed up the skin with a friction-glove, ampoules containing thyroid hormone with or without the addition of an enzyme are rubbed in with the palm of the hand. The course consists of thirty to forty ampoules; a single ampoule is applied daily, six days a week, to one side on even days, to the other on odd days. The only drawback, for those women who like the atmosphere and accoutrements of the modern clinic, is that self-treatment is rather a lonely occupation. Otherwise, its results are nearly always as good as those obtained by more sophisticated techniques, and just as lasting.

The improvement, usually apparent after a couple of weeks, will last for several months, or even a year or two in particularly favourable circumstances. But a relapse is inevitable and the whole process must be repeated from the beginning.

Various means have been suggested whereby these remedies can be made more effective and their benefits longer lasting: among them, 'ultrasonics' and electrical stimulation, both of which stimulate the circulation and provoke rhythmic contractions of the muscular mass in the treated area. They do have some effect, but it is relatively weak.

There is no doubt, however, that a re-education of the muscles helps to maintain the improvement.

MASSAGE

For this reason massage too has its uses, provided that it is correctly applied: *any form of brutal pummelling must be strictly avoided*. It horrifies me to hear of sessions more like all-in-wrestling than massage, during which, under the pretence of kneading, the 'cellulitic' mass is crushed to a pulp with the bare hands. This can only result in the destruction, once and for all, of the distended, fragile connective fibres and the formation of a soggy mass of jelly and ruptured fat cells: a straightforward case of 'cellulite' is consequently transformed into a contused mass, marbled with bruises, and, worst of all, the network of capillary vessels in the dermis is so badly damaged that it becomes visible in the shape of broken veins.

When correctly applied, on the other hand, by using stroking, rubbing, and vibrations, massage helps to improve the pitted, orange-peel look, stimulate local circulation and the elimination of waste products by the cells, and tone up the musculature.

SPORT

Nothing is better for muscular re-education than sport. Riding is particularly effective, but some people are either afraid of horses or else, for reasons of age or practicability, unable to join a riding-school.

In their case, I advise walking — at a brisker pace than for the purpose of losing weight, up and down hill if possible — and bicycling, which is excellent exercise for 'cellulite'.

One scarcely heard any mention of 'cellulite' during the Occupation, among that generation who lived in Paris during the last war and got to know the city through the use of their legs: you don't notice the hills in a car, but there are uphill slopes everywhere. Downhill slopes too, of course, but you don't remember those. It's the uphill treks that you remember: from the Gare Saint-Lazare to the Place Clichy, from the Place de la Concorde or the Trocadéro to the Étoile. You might think that, thirty years later, you could exercise your muscles on foot or on a bicycle at less risk to your life than in those days. No such luck! Cars have replaced machine guns and the risk is as great as ever.

'STRETCH-MARKS'

If the treatment of 'cellulite' is fraught with uncertainty, that of 'stretch-marks' is non-existent.

No doctor likes to be confronted with a situation which he is helpless to remedy. Whenever this happens, his *raison d'être*, to heal and alleviate suffering, is called into question. It grieves him to have to tell a young woman, in despair because her stomach is disfigured by ugly strips of atrophied skin, that he can do nothing for her.

As everyone knows, the commonest cause of 'stretch-marks' is pregnancy. Seventy-five per cent of women develop them by about the sixth month. The striations can be long or short, between half a centimetre and a centimetre wide, and are satin-like, puckered and mauvish-pink in colour. They are unalterable from the moment they appear: only their colour will gradually fade to white. They can also occur at puberty or in the course of serious infectious diseases, such as typhoid, and they have been observed in concentration-camp survivors.

It's always the junction of the limbs with the torso and the torso itself which are affected. The 'stretch-marks' radiate outwards from the nipples, downwards from the hips and on the stomach, sideways across the lumbar region and obliquely across the shoulders. They result from the destruction of the network of elastic fibres of the dermis – the reason for their scarred, puckered appearance – and are commonly supposed to be a purely feminine affliction, caused by the skin being stretched in some way. Both these suppositions are incorrect.

For one thing, *so-called 'stretch-marks' are not uncommon in men*; and for another, a young person's skin can be stretched to the limit without the elastic fibres being ruptured. However, it is precisely in young people that they are most often seen. There are good grounds for believing that they are due to the action of the cortisone secreted by the suprarenal glands: certainly, there is increased activity in these glands during the last months of pregnancy, and frequently at the onset of puberty; certain diseases where the suprarenal glands produce too much cortisone are also accompanied by 'stretch-marks'; and treatments involving strong doses of cortisone can also provoke them. Altogether, there are an impressive number of arguments consistent with this theory.

But the fact that we have hit upon their likely cause does not mean that we are able to cure them, for any degeneration of the elastic tissue is irreparable. When an ordinary piece of elastic perishes, we throw it away and buy a new one. Unfortunately, when the elastic bands of the skin 'perish', we can neither throw them away nor replace them. Even cosmetic surgery cannot help.

The only hope is to prevent them from developing in the first place. So far, however, preventive treatment has come up against insuperable obstacles: the only way to slow down the secretion of the suprarenal glands is by using cortisone derivatives and these, as we have seen, present certain grave risks. There can be no question of using them blindly, least of all during pregnancy, in order to prevent a condition which may never materialise. To replace one risk, that of purely aesthetic damage, by another, far more serious one, is never justified.

Gynaecologists frequently advise their patients to massage themselves with vitamin-based preparations or preparations containing amniotic fluid, the fluid in which the embryo is suspended; (during labour, the amniotic membrane ruptures and the fluid escapes: this is what is called 'breaking the waters').

Well, at least it can't do any harm ...

DISORDERS OF THE ADNEXAL TISSUES

There are four special formations 'annexed' to the skin: the nails and hair, which form part of its protective mechanism and also serve to ornament it; the sebaceous glands and the sweat glands.

I don't propose to discuss the nails in this book; their frequent, numerous and complicated fluctuations in health are a highly specialised field of dermatology; while they tend to reflect the general physical condition, their appearance is simply a question of manicure and presents no special problems.

The same cannot be said of perspiration and the hair; disorders of one or the other can affect to a considerable degree the best-formed of bodies and the most attractive of faces.

PERSPIRATION

All human beings perspire, and a certain degree of perspiration is essential if the organism is to maintain its proper equilibrium.

As we have seen, in the context of problems of skin hydration, insensible perspiration amounts to between 400–600 grams of water a day. This rate of elimination is constant and even greater than that of the lungs, which gives some idea of its importance.

Apart from certain special circumstances, such as fever, a rise in external temperature or a heightening of the emotions, all of which may cause it to vary both in degree and duration, it is one of our fundamental methods of salt-excretion. As long as we perspire at the normal rate, perspiration is not an embarrassing phenomenon. But for some people, its copiousness and odour amount almost to physical disability.

Although the effects of perspiration do not strictly speaking constitute skin damage, I believe they come within the compass of this book if only because beauty is surely the art of making oneself attractive to others; and not merely attractive to look at, but also attractive to touch and to smell; and no matter how beautiful you are, you won't be attractive if you smell unpleasant.

Moreover, the problems of sweat and its odours are closely linked to those of skin hygiene, not to say hygiene in general, which gives me a chance to say a few words on the subject.

THE SWEAT GLANDS

There are two sorts of glands which secrete sweat: first, those glands scattered over the entire surface of the skin: between two and three million of them. They are especially numerous on the forehead, the soles of the feet and the palms of the hands, where over a thousand per square centimetre have been counted.

These are the eccrine glands; their secretion is higher in men than in women and diminishes progressively with age in both sexes.

They don't all secrete at once, but in groups, taking it in turns so that the group which has just been active can rest while a neighbouring group takes over. Both the order of activity and the number of groups functioning at any one time increases with heat, physical exercise and emotional stress; an increase of half a degree in the internal temperature will also send them into action.

As I explained earlier, in people with seborrhea the sweat plays a part in the diffusion of the sebum which spreads more rapidly on the surface of the skin when this is damp: skin looks oilier when there is little sebum and a lot of sweat than when there is more sebum and less sweat.

Alongside the eccrine glands, in the armpits, the genital region, the nostrils and on the nipples, there are 'apocrine' glands which differ from them profoundly in every way.

The pore, invisible to the naked eye, through which the eccrine glands deposit the sweat on the surface of the skin, is quite distinct from the pore of the sebaceous glands; the apocrine gland, on the

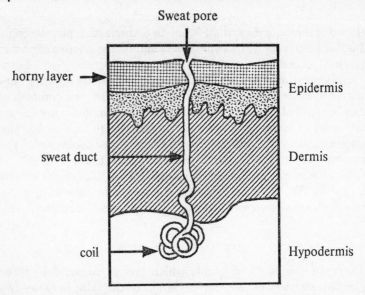

DIAGRAM III   The sweat gland

The sweat secreted by the coil traverses the dermis and epidermis by means of the excretory canal and flows out at the surface of the skin.

other hand, opens into the hair-sheath and thus its secretion is eliminated through the same pore as the sebum; eccrine sweat is exuded in drops, whereas apocrine sweat is exuded in the form of a glutinous milky substance which solidifies when dry.

Whereas the eccrine glands are already functioning in childhood, the apocrine glands develop only at puberty; they are more numerous and begin to secrete earlier in women than in men; their secretion is augmented just before menstruation and diminished by pregnancy.

Lastly, they respond more to nervous, sexual and emotional stimulation than to variations in temperature. They react to stimulation within fifteen seconds, but after discharging they become passive and cannot secrete for several hours.

In those people who sweat copiously at the slightest provocation, it isn't the apocrine glands which are responsible. Despite the fact that the armpits are rich in apocrine glands, the liquid that flows out, staining our clothes, is eccrine, not apocrine, sweat.

For some people, perspiration can become a truly unbearable nightmare. Their hands are not merely damp, they are drenched.

Everything they touch is stained or moistened; they are virtually excluded from certain professions, such as dressmaking, leather-working, clockmaking, bookbinding or draughtsmanship. Sweaty feet, which usually go with sweaty hands, rot their shoes and socks. Their perpetually damp epidermis takes on a spongy, greyish, un-healthy look. They will suddenly pour with sweat from head to foot, to the point where they need to mop themselves with a towel. Some people sweat in a particular place, always the same one, such as the jaw, or, when eating, the lower half of the face.

It wouldn't be so bad if this 'hyperidrosis' didn't smell, but its odour can be literally foetid. It predominates in the armpits, the feet and occasionally the groin, and is due to the decomposition of the saturated, spongy epidermis brought about by the bacteria present on the surface of the skin.

This repulsive smell should not be confused with the smell of apocrine sweat. Although this always has a slight smell, generally stronger in redheaded people than others, it is only offensive when decomposed by bacteria and not normally disagreeable; it's even thought to play a part in sexual behaviour and attraction; from this point of view, therefore, the excessive use of deodorants and perfumes would seem undesirable.

In this, as in everything else, we should keep a sense of propor-tion and not equate our bodily hygiene with the hygienic processes applied to the sort of foodstuffs which come sealed in plastic bags, guaranteed germ-free and ready to eat.

Generally speaking, most people need do no more than observe regularly a few basic rules of cleanliness, such as a daily wash all over with a good plain white soap. Anyone who finds it incredible that I should even bother to point this out hasn't had a doctor's experience of the dirtiness of human beings: it has to be seen to be believed!

I know, and my colleagues know, that soap and water are only too readily replaced by deodorants, and that immaculate make-up and elegantly varnished nails are nothing to go by. Beware of re-moving that nail-polish, if you don't want to reveal nails ringed with dirt and which have clearly never seen a nail-brush!

Beware of examining that make-up too closely, of peering into the ears or lifting up the hair, if you don't appreciate the effects of contrast: on some necks I've seen you could draw graffiti, white on grey, with a cotton-tipped stick dipped in spirit.

Every mother knows that fourteen- or fifteen-year-old boys have a rooted aversion to soap and water. At that age, you don't wash if you can possibly avoid it. But it's nothing to worry about: they usually get over it as soon as they meet a girl they want to impress. But when it continues into adulthood, it closely resembles what the psychoanalysts call infantile regression, a state in which the adult remains fixed in attitudes normal in childhood, but abnormal in grown-ups.

Hygiene comes before beauty, before embellishment. Looking after our skin doesn't simply mean covering up the visible bits with various cosmetics in order to protect it and make it look pretty. And the first thing to do is to wash both what shows and what doesn't show.

In these days of environmental pollution, it is not just the rivers and oceans which become contaminated, but also our skin. If we are to keep our epidermis in good condition, it's every bit as important to rid it of pollutants as it is to keep it balanced and protected with creams and lotions.

Sophisticated aids are quite unnecessary: even people who don't bother to wash know that soap and water are all that you need. As for the brand of soap you choose, the main thing to remember is never to use cheap soaps which might prove to be irritants. Whether you are a man or a woman, if you have a normal skin you can't do better than use a traditional plain white soap.

But if your epidermis is very dried up, super-fatted soap, pharmaceutical soap, or one of those preparations containing lipoproteins that don't damage the chemical substances in the horny layer can be helpful.

In the case of men who do particularly dirty jobs, such pharmaceutical and liquid soaps may be used on the face. Otherwise, a rinse with a face-flannel soaked in clear cold water after shaving is quite sufficient. Moreover, cold water is an excellent decongestive 'after-shave' lotion.

As I've already explained at length in the preceding chapters, women should never use soap on their faces: they are much more delicate than men's. Every now and then, someone will cite the case of her eighty-five-year-old grandmother who has washed her face in soap and water night and morning all her life and whose skin is the envy of all. I don't deny that such lucky women exist. But they are the exception that proves the rule, and the rule is that very few women's faces can stand up to such treatment for long. A good cleansing milk, correctly used, cleans just as well as soap, and there is no point in tempting fate.

After washing or bathing, the skin must be carefully dried, especially in the folds beneath the breasts, the crotch, under the arms and between the toes, in order to prevent the maceration that encourages bacteria to breed. It's a good idea to powder these areas with a talc: the folds of the skin have a natural tendency to dampness which can be counteracted by the absorbent and drying properties of talcum powder.

Deodorisers, or 'deodorants', can be useful when there is dampness in the folds of the skin, which is likely to cause bacteriological fermentation. They have no effect whatever on perspiration itself, which can only be treated by medicine or surgery, but the antiseptic they contain prevents fermentation by destroying the bacteria. Occasionally a deodorant will provoke an allergic reaction in the form of blotches and itching which will clear up as soon as you stop using it.

These elementary principles of hygiene are adequate and valid for everyone. But it is just as bad for the skin to overdo them as it is to neglect them: the sort of cleanliness fanatic who baths twice a day using harsh detergents in the water, scrubbing herself until she is raw and rinsing her face with alcohol-based lotions is likely to ruin her skin even more quickly than the person who doesn't wash at all.

Of course, the skin must be kept clean; but there's no need to exaggerate, and damage to the horny layer, its first line of defence, should be avoided above all. Bubble-baths are among the worst offenders; by all means amuse yourself with one occasionally, but don't be led astray by all that pure-looking white foam — after using one of these products in the bath you won't have to clean it or call in the plumber to unblock the drain: all will be clear, clean, scoured, polished, shining, including your skin, which will take far less kindly to such treatment.

THE HAIR

When describing the different parts of the skin at the beginning of this book, I deliberately made no more than a passing reference to hair, in order to avoid overburdening a chapter already somewhat dry and indigestible. But if we are to understand the life-cycle of this important formation extruding from the skin, we must first know something about its composition.

THE STRUCTURE OF THE HAIR

The hair is composed of keratin, a modified version of the same keratin which forms the horny layer of the skin.

Hairs are rooted in the skin within a finger-shaped sheath called the 'follicle'. The wall of this sheath is formed by a fold in the epidermis which extends downwards through the skin into the hypodermis.

At its nearest point to the cutaneous surface, the upper part of the follicle forms a duct, the 'follicular canal', in which the hair stands free: this section of the hair is called the 'shaft'. Since the sebaceous duct also opens into the follicular canal, the hair shaft emerges through the same pore which secretes the sebum: this ensures its direct lubrication.

In the lower part of the follicle, the follicular wall and the hair are fused. This entire section of the hair constitutes its root, the deepest part of which is known as the 'bulb'.

The hair is not a simple filament: it has an extremely complex structure the details of which I shall not go into here. Suffice it to say that it consists, broadly speaking, of a central cortex surrounded by several protective layers. The hair contains neither nerves nor blood-vessels; clearly, therefore, there is none of the so-called 'sap', disappointing though this may be to those who say—and I have heard them—that dull, limp hair is the result of escaping 'sap' and that all you need to do, in order to strengthen the hair, is to stop the leak by singeing the ends. It's a charming idea; unfortunately there's not a word of truth in it.

DIFFERENT TYPES OF HAIR

There are very many different types of hair which, in one form or another, cover almost the entire surface of the skin, with the exception of the palms of the hands and the soles of the feet.

Hair differs considerably in volume, structure and colour depending on race and on the individual.

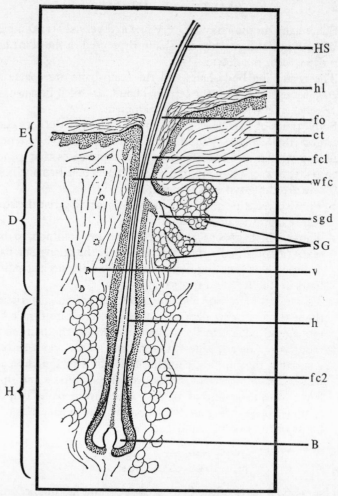

DIAGRAM IV: Vertical section of a hair follicle with its hair and its sebaceous gland

   E: epidermis (with its horny layer (hl) indented into the follicular canal which it has a tendency to obstruct
   D: dermis (with its blood vessels (v) and its connective tissue (ct)
   H: hypodermis (with fat cells (fc2))
  HS: hair (h) shaft emerging from the skin through the follicular opening (fo)
 fc1: follicular canal
 wfc: wall of follicular canal formed by the indentation of the epidermis which is depressed into the hypodermis
   B: hair bulb
  SG: sebaceous gland with duct (sgd) opening into hair follicle

Some hairs on the body are very fine and very short; compared to other types of hair, they are shallowly rooted in the skin: hairs like these form the down.

The remaining body-hairs and the scalp-hairs are coarse and deeply-rooted: these are the terminal hairs, so-called because they have reached the limit of their development.

Some types of hair are straight, others wavy, yet others curly; whatever their colour — fair, brown, black or red — they tend to fade and whiten at some stage, later in some cases than others; eventually, towards the end of life, everyone's hair turns white.

There are three types of terminal hairs:

1 Those present from infancy in both boys and girls: the scalp-hair, eyebrows and eyelashes;

2 Those which appear at puberty and are common to both sexes (ambosexual): the underarm hair, the triangular patch of pubic hair pointing down towards the sex organ, and the hairs on the legs and forearms;

3 The sexual hairs, so-called because they are characteristic of the male sex, being dependent on the secretion of male hormone, and not normally present in women: the hairs in the moustache, beard, side-whiskers, ears, nose, on the back, encircling the nipples, covering the centre of the chest in a mat which sometimes extends over the shoulders and upper back, forming a line of varying width from navel to pubic triangle, or growing in tufts between the buttocks, on the backs of the thighs, hands and feet.

THE LIFE-CYCLE OF HAIR

All hairs on all parts of the body grow, rest and fall out according to a cycle which is repeated uninterruptedly throughout life: a hair continues to grow as long as the cells lying at the base of the follicle which produce it maintain their high rate of activity; when this activity suddenly ceases, the hair, instead of falling out immediately, remains attached by the root until the new hair destined to replace it gradually pushes it upwards through the follicular duct on the 'I'm the King of the Castle' principle.

The duration of the life-cycle varies from one part of the body to another: in the case of the eyebrows and eyelashes, it is between 140 and 150 days; in the case of the beard, between 7 and 11 months and even as long as 36 months; in the case of the armpits, about 7 months. The scalp-hair has the longest life-cycle of all: some people put it at four years, others five or even seven.

The periods of growth and rest vary according to the location of the hair on the body. In the pubic region in women, for example, they are almost the same: from 11 to 18 months of growth, followed by 12 to 17 months of rest. The eyebrows and eyelashes, on the other hand, have a very short growing period lasting between 30 and 40 days, and a very long resting period lasting 105 days.

The reverse is true of the hair on the head, where the period of rest — about two to three months — is extremely brief when compared to the period of active growth.

Hair grows fastest during the warm season, when men often have to shave twice a day in order to look presentable, whereas once a day in winter is enough.

Hair-growth also differs between the sexes: women's hair grows faster than men's — between 10·2 and 10·8 millimetres and 9·3 and 10·2 millimetres a month respectively.

The speed of growth slows down with age: the period of most rapid growth occurs between the ages of fifteen and thirty; between fifty and sixty it slows down markedly; in the case of the beard and armpits, this slowing-down process is delayed until the age of sixty-five; but the eyebrows and pubic hair maintain the same rate of growth throughout life.

As for the effect of the seasons on falling hair, it has not yet been scientifically proved whether or not human beings moult like animals from the head and body. The prevailing opinion is that hair falls out more or less regularly throughout the year.

This background information goes some way to meet the constantly recurring questions from those people — and there are an increasing number of them — who are anxious about their hair in general and their scalp hair in particular.

The facts explain, for example, why there is never any immediate relationship between hair-loss and its cause. I'm often being told: 'I had terrible indigestion a couple of weeks ago, doctor, and my hair has been coming out in handfuls ever since.'

If so, it's pure coincidence: for one thing, no one has yet lost hair through indigestion — or a liver attack, come to that — and then, even if this were possible, there would be a delay of eight

M

to twelve weeks; in other words, the duration of the inactive period which preceded the condemned hair's expulsion by its successor. *In the case of abnormal hair-loss, you need to go back two or three months to find its likely cause.*

If we stick to the facts there is no risk of our mistaking normal hair-loss for a disorder, or of becoming needlessly alarmed when, after the menopause, the hair no longer grows as fast as it used to; this doesn't mean that there's anything the matter with the hair, or that one is about to go bald – it's a natural phenomenon, common to all human beings.

Any type of hair disorder, whether to the body hair or the scalp hair, adversely affects our looks; and all types of hair disorder are diseases in the strict sense of the word.

Two in particular concern us all. Because of their prevalence and the anxiety they cause, what amounts to an industry, extremely lucrative at that, has grown up around them, in which ignorance and credulity are matched only by the most blatant charlatanism. I'm referring, of course, to the abnormal development of body-hair known as 'hirsutism' and the types of hair loss known as 'alopecia' and baldness.

HIRSUTISM

Hirsutism is a condition where the development of body hair is exaggerated. In a man it is not a disease but simply an exaggeration of normal hair growth, *whereas in a woman it is always abnormal.*

THE HIRSUTE MALE

Some men are entirely covered with a veritable fleece from their shoulders to their ankles, associated in the popular mind with the idea of virility, even though in reality this is not necessarily the case.

FEMININE HIRSUTISM

But in the case of a woman, this unwanted hair poses real problems, whether she really has an exaggerated amount of body hair or merely imagines that she has. If the latter, there is a real danger that she herself may bring about a condition known as 'hypertrichosis' through her own ill-judged efforts.

Hypertrichosis is an exclusively feminine disease and consists of an abnormal development of terminal hairs on a hairless part of the body; by hairless, I mean a part of the body where you would normally expect to find only a fine down: the presence of down is normal on the cheeks and upper lip of a woman, that of terminal hairs is not.

Hypertrichosis may either be localised, in the form of a hairy mole, for instance, or widespread. It can exist in infancy – some babies have a thick, woolly growth on the forearms which should be ignored as it will soon disappear – and it can also develop at any time of life, whether from internal or external causes.

THE EXTERNAL CAUSES OF HYPERTRICHOSIS

There are two possible external causes: treatment involving male hormones and treatment involving mechanical depilation.*

The male hormone or its derivatives are often prescribed for gynaecological reasons. They constitute the classic treatment for fibromas, heavy or painful periods, and the swelling of the breasts accompanied by the formation of hard, sensitive cysts. If a woman receiving this treatment is *predisposed* to hypertrichosis, she may notice a change in her body hair, especially on the chin and upper lip where the down will gradually be supplanted by terminal hairs. Not all women react in this way, of course; some can take male hormones, even over a prolonged period, without growing hairs. But there is no way of knowing what your reaction will be until you have tried, so, unless it is really necessary, it's better not to put it to the test.

When used on the legs, a wax depilatory will not lead to the development of hypertrichosis; in fact, if repeated often enough, this method leads to the eventual disappearance of the hairs.

But, without our knowing why, the precise opposite applies to the face: any form of mechanical depilation is far and away the chief cause of hypertrichosis of the chin and upper lip. The results are worse when wax is used because it strips off the down indiscriminately, unlike tweezers.

As the beauty-salons proliferate, so do the number of women

* There are three recognised methods of depilation: mechanical, by means of tweezers or wax; chemical, by means of depilatory pastes; electrical, by means of coagulation of the hair-root. (A-B)

who become slaves to the virtual moustache and 'beard' of tough, prickly hairs which are the result of using such methods over the years.

The drama usually unfolds in five acts:

Act One : Mary, catching sight of herself in a particular light, or examining herself in a magnifying mirror (which distorts reality by exaggerating it), sees a faint shadow on her upper lip. Had she been a blonde she wouldn't even have noticed it, but as she's very dark something can just be seen, even if only from certain angles.

Act Two : She makes an appointment at the beauty-salon. The well-meaning but ignorant beauty-consultant doesn't shrink from her task. 'We'll soon fix that,' she says confidently. She warms a little wax, spreads it over the offending down with the skill born of practice, then strips it off with a short, sharp tug: 'There you are! That's all there is to it, look how smooth and clean your upper lip is now … '

Act Three : Three weeks to a month later, the down has re-grown. Mary returns to the beauty-salon where the treatment is repeated; and so it goes on, without apparent ill-effect. It seems quite simple: as the down reappears, you have it stripped off. All goes well until the day when that tiresome down seems more noticeable. One could swear that it was growing faster, getting thicker, that there was more of it than before. Now the depilations must be done more often, and they are becoming more and more unpleasant; the thicker the down, the harder it is to pull out. But it has to be done — one can't go about looking like that.

Act Four : The down has finally disappeared for good; it took a few years to achieve this, but it has come about at last. Instead, there's a splendid growth of strong healthy hairs which have to be removed one by one with the tweezers as they prick their way through the skin; wax doesn't work any longer, the hair is too coarse. It means a good ten minutes' work in front of the mirror every day, and it leaves behind red patches, often aggravated by little spots: the repeated extraction of deep-rooted hairs is a con-siderable irritant.

Act Five : At the dermatologist's. He casts an eye over the battle-field: the skin is speckled with dark hairs poking through the epidermis. Others, just beneath the surface, give the skin a greyish tinge. There are red marks here and there, the vestiges of pustules which, needless to say, have been squeezed. Next, he runs his finger over the skin: it feels like a rasp. Finally he asks:

'How old are you?'

'Thirty.'

'How long have you been using depilatories?'

'Oh, I've almost forgotten, about ten years.'

'Does your mother have the same trouble?'

'No, not at all.'

'Do you have sisters?'

'Yes, one older sister; she doesn't suffer from it either.'

'Tell me, do you have any other hairs like these on your body: on your breasts, around the nipples, between your breasts or on your stomach leading up to the navel?'

THE INTERNAL CAUSES OF HYPERTRICHOSIS

This is a very important question; it's not at all uncommon for a woman who comes for treatment for facial hypertrichosis to be suffering in reality from what we call 'male-pattern hirsutes', in which case the hairs which worry her because they show are part of a more widespread condition that she hasn't mentioned, either because she is shy or because it hasn't occurred to her.

Male-pattern hirsutes denotes the presence of secondary male sexual characteristics in women: for example, underdeveloped or shrinking breasts, an enlarged clitoris, menstruation becomes irregular or ceases altogether, there is a drop in pitch of the voice, or a modification of the subcutaneous fat which alters the shape of the body.

Body hair is yet another of these secondary sexual characteristics and male-pattern hirsutes is the development of those hairs I mentioned earlier, the 'sexual hairs' normally found in men.

Unlike the hairs on the chin and upper-lip, these hairs are only embarrassing to women when they are wearing a bathing-suit, in which case they can simply be shaved off. Nevertheless, they are highly significant because, unlike the hairs on the chin or the upper lip which may be the result of unwise depilations *they are all spontaneous*; moreover, in a considerable number of cases, they result from glandular trouble: hair, like the sebaceous gland, is a focal point for the male hormone, and everything that I have said in connection with its role in seborrhea applies equally here. In fact, male-pattern hirsutes is quite often associated with acne.

In cases of true male-pattern hirsutes, therefore, the first thing to be done is to have analyses made of the hormones present in the urine and, if necessary, the blood, *especially where there is a combination of menstrual disorders and seborrhea*. The precision of these analyses gives extremely reliable results. Some laboratories specialise in this type of work: laboratories, like doctors, tend to specialise more and more as research requires out-of-the-ordinary techniques and equipment, as in this case.

It can thus be established first of all whether or not there is any hormonal disorder: women of certain races – the natives of those countries along the Mediterranean seaboard for instance – are often very hairy, *constitutionally*, from mother to daughter, without there being any over-secretion of male hormones. The mere fact that it has been clinically established that a masculine-type hair-growth is present does not automatically mean that there is also a glandular disorder.

However, if the disorder exists, one can then discover its precise origins. This is important because the treatment will vary according to whether it is the ovaries or the suprarenal glands which are misbehaving.

Lastly, by means of periodic tests made during the course of treatment, we can monitor its effects and make minute adjustments where necessary, all of which amounts to a guarantee of effectiveness and safety for the patient.

THE TREATMENT OF HIRSUTISM

The down may diminish in response to the appropriate internal treatment, but *never the terminal hairs*: there is no exception to this rule. Consequently, *the sole method of getting rid of unwanted terminal hairs once and for all is to destroy them by means of electrolysis*.

Even this method only works properly when the hypertrichosis is stable, such as when it has been caused by mechanical depilation or when it's constitutional in origin.

When hirsutism is glandular in origin the results of electrolysis are very undependable because, due to the constant stimulation of the male hormone, new hairs go on developing in the place of the hairs just removed. The process becomes never-ending.

'Is that why people say that electrolysis doesn't work?' Mary may ask at this point.

'Partly. The effects of electrolysis can indeed be nullified if the doctor hasn't taken the trouble to regulate the secretion of male hormones correctly, where this was necessary. Sometimes it can be the fault of a clumsy operator. When properly carried out it is a very effective and reliable method, but it must be combined with the appropriate treatment where necessary and applied with due skill.'

'How is it done?'

'It's quite straightforward: one uses very fine needles and a weak current, as in the treatment of broken veins, and one inserts the point of the needle into the hair-bulb so as to destroy the zone where the hair grows.'

'Is it painful?'

'No, but it tickles; and some places are more sensitive than others: the upper lip, for instance, and the neck. Most people find it perfectly bearable. Now and then one comes across a patient who is rather apprehensive and makes a bit of a fuss ... '

'How can you tell if you've reached the bulb?'

'The hair should come out easily when you remove it with tweezers. If it resists, you have missed the bulb. It mustn't be pulled out but re-treated.'

'I see, but what I really meant to ask was how can you be sure that you're putting the needle into the right place?'

'By following the direction of the hair-shaft with the needle.'

'So you need to be able to see the hair?'

'Exactly. *A woman who wants to have electrolysis should never pluck her hairs herself*. This is not to say that she must let them grow long – just a millimetre or two. She can cut them with a pair of sharp scissors as necessary.'

'But that's awful! One would look an absolute fright ... '

'I agree that it needs considerable determination to go around for weeks or even months with the equivalent of two days' growth of beard. But there's no alternative: take it or leave it.'

'Why should it take months?'

'It all depends on the number of hairs to be treated. One can remove 100, sometimes 150, in the course of one half-hour session. But a woman who has been plucking her down with tweezers can easily have up to 1,500 hairs, and I've counted over 10,000 on a patient who, like you, had been using a wax depilatory for ten years. I ought to add that she also had a very high secretion of male hormone from her ovaries: the combination of mechanical depilation and hormonal stimulation was disastrous: she was obliged to shave.'

'How often can one have it done?'

'One should leave eight to ten days before going over the same area again. The skin needs time to recover between sessions.'

'Why? Is the skin inflamed?'

'A little. Minute scabs form at each puncture point. This is unavoidable, although the needles, apart from their point, are covered in insulating material. But it's nothing to worry about; the tiny scabs fall off in a week at the most. You mustn't pick at them, of course.'

'Do they leave scars?'

'No, providing that one doesn't do too much at once – that is, try and depilate an area completely. The puncture points should be well spaced out over a wide area. If they are made too close together, the tiny cauterisations tend to merge, forming one large cauterised area which then leaves a scar.

'When it is done correctly, depilation leaves no trace, or only minuscule marks that most patients gladly accept in return for the pleasure of getting rid of their detested hairs.

'Nevertheless, there are circumstances in which visible traces may remain no matter how careful one is: when treating the upper lip, where one must use a very light touch and only coagulate a few hairs at a time and when treating down. These hairs being only shallowly rooted, there is a greater risk of burning the surface of the skin than with deeper-rooted hairs; it is therefore better to leave them alone. Women who ask to have their down removed should be refused: when it's fair, it should be left alone, when it's dark, it should be bleached.

'To sum up, electrolysis should be used only on terminal hairs which can be permanently destroyed with satisfactory results.

'These can be equally satisfactory on the chest and stomach; together with the face, these are the only areas of the body where it is unquestionably worth doing.

'Obviously there is nothing to stop people having it done on their arms and legs. It seems madness to me. But if the idea is to exploit the customer rather than treat a patient, why not, after all?'

CHANGES AND DISORDERS AFFECTING THE SCALP AND HAIR

I've already made it clear that the properties claimed for cosmetic creams, milks and lotions bear little or no relation to their actual value.

But when it comes to fooling the public, the cosmetic manufacturers can't hold a candle to the charlatans who are in business to 'treat' hair. What's more, they fool the public at its own expense; it's so lucrative a business that they don't hesitate to risk prosecution. A fine is a drop in the ocean compared to their profits, and if they are closed down they merely open up again under another name.

As the law stands there is nothing to prevent anyone from setting up a 'hair clinic' or, even more outrageously, as a 'hair specialist' or 'trichologist'. Admittedly even if it doesn't mean anything, the word 'trichology' has a scientific ring, all the better to impress the client.

Whatever they call themselves, the methods of such practitioners are all the same: a few hairs are taken from the scalp and examined with scientific-looking apparatus in front of the client. This rigmarole is an important part of the scene-setting. Next, a form is filled up, in order to make it all look respectable, and lastly, of course, a diagnosis is made whose sole object is to induce the client to embark on a course of 'treatment' the results of which are guaranteed ... guaranteed, that is, to pay off the cost of the equipment and the overheads in double-quick time!

As a rule, these courses involve a series of twelve 'treatments' payable in advance – possibly costing £100 or more which cannot be recovered under any insurance scheme – together with various products to be used at home and, naturally enough, supplied by the enterprise concerned. Their contents are a secret, mind you! – but since they are completely useless, it doesn't matter.

The most extraordinary aspect of the whole business, when you come to think of it, is not that charlatans like these exist and that they should extract as much money as they can from people who entrust themselves to them, but that there should be such an enormous number of people who are naïve, credulous and ignorant enough to believe in them.

In my experience, men know perfectly well that no one has yet discovered any sure way of preventing baldness. When they consult a doctor, it's not because they're under any illusions about going bald, but because they want to know what likelihood there is in their case, or if by any chance some new way has been discovered of slowing down the process; when you tell them that all existing methods are useless, they seldom seem surprised.

The only other explanation is that people go to a trichologist as they go to a faith-healer, in search of a miracle.

Unfortunately, where hair is concerned, miracles don't happen; there are no examples of bald pates miraculously garnished with hair, or treatments which can prevent hair from falling out as much or as little as nature intended.

Hair-loss may be temporary or permanent.

Temporary hair-loss is known as 'alopecia', permanent hair-loss as baldness.

The most typical form of alopecia is the hair-loss — sometimes massive and alarming — that follows childbirth or a disease accompanied by high fever, such as influenza, pneumonia or typhoid.

I am quite accustomed to seeing women arrive in my consulting rooms at the end of their tether, holding out envelopes stuffed with that morning's hair-combings as dramatic proof of their wretchedness. It turns out that two or three months previously they had given birth to a bouncing eight-pound baby, and that everything had gone quite normally. I never have any trouble in reassuring them: this type of alopecia always clears up of its own accord and their hair will grow again as good as new.

MASCULINE BALDNESS

The hair-loss which leads to baldness is seldom so spectacular. It is far more deceptive and insidious, taking years before it denudes the scalp completely. Moreover, there is no relationship whatever between the proportion of hair lost daily and the rate of progress of the baldness; everything depends on the ratio between what falls out and what grows in its place.

Normal hair-loss in a man without thinning hair is estimated at between 20 and 30 hairs a day.

And yet some men can lose as many as 50, 80 or 100 hairs a day, or even more, without there being any thinning of the hair because the loss is regularly replaced by an equivalent growth.

On the other hand, there are men who go bald while losing only

15 to 20 hairs a day, or less than the normal amount; but in their case the loss is only partially compensated for by new growth.

In other words, baldness results from a permanent deficit. As long as you make as much as you lose, you maintain a healthy bank balance; should expenditure exceed income, however, the result is bankruptcy.

The onset of baldness follows a characteristic pattern: typically, the first signs appear at the age of eighteen in men, affecting the frontal zone at the summit of the forehead and the crown of the head. The hairline begins to recede at the temples.

But a receding hairline means nothing in itself: the way the hair grows on the forehead is a secondary sexual characteristic and, in boys after puberty, the hairline recedes in the form of a capital M, the uprights following the outline of the temples and the oblique strokes that of the 'peak'.

In girls the hairline normally remains unbroken, following the line of the temples in the shape of an upside-down U. For a woman, therefore, unlike a man, a receding hairline is a bad omen for the future.

The direst symptom for a man is the thinning and then receding of the frontal zone. This occurs in waves, interspersed with periods when the process appears to have come to a halt. But with each succeeding wave, the area of depleted surface is enlarged, and the growing hairs — for hairs continue to grow throughout this relentless progress towards baldness — become fewer and fewer, finer and finer, until all that remains is a circlet of hair, which persists throughout life, surrounding a scalp sparsely covered in fine down with, here and there, a single hair that for some reason has escaped.

The rate of progress towards baldness in men varies considerably. Some men are completely bald by the time they are twenty-five years old; in others the final blow doesn't happen until they are in their thirties.

Apart from this classic type of baldness, known as 'Hippocratic' baldness because Hippocrates, the father of medicine, suffered from it, there are the conditions of partial and delayed baldness.

In partial baldness, a single zone only is affected; either the crown, to a greater or lesser extent, or the frontal zone, which is denuded, pushing the limits of the hair back to the centre of the cranium.

In delayed baldness, the hair begins to fall out at the age of thirty or later; it takes the form of thinning to a greater or lesser degree but seldom results in the complete baldness which follows from premature hair-loss.

BALDNESS IN WOMEN

Baldness in women is very different in appearance. Alopecia is the usual name for it, rather than baldness, because in the case of women the hair-loss is not necessarily irremediable and irreversible except when it results from the kind of hair-style known as the 'pony-tail'.

The 'pony-tail' can lead to irreversible baldness along the hair-line, because the forehead and temples are the zones where the traction exerted on the hair-shaft is greatest. This continuous traction causes circulatory disorders in the blood-vessels which nourish the hair-root, which in turn degenerates.

This disorder is frequently observed in Eskimo women who traditionally wear their hair in a pony-tail, and for some years after the last war there was a virtual epidemic of it in Western Europe which caused this otherwise delightful fashion to be quickly abandoned.

As a rule, hair-loss in women leads either to widespread alopecia affecting the whole head, involving thinning to a greater or lesser degree, or a form of alopecia affecting the temples only: the very zone, interestingly enough, which is never affected in men. This is one of many unexplained peculiarities.

'Hippocratic' baldness does not occur in women, except at a very advanced age.

As in men, hair-loss in women may start early, between the ages of seventeen and nineteen, or be delayed. On the whole, early loss signifies a widespread alopecia and is especially distressing, since those afflicted know in advance that their hair will always be a problem, to some extent, for the rest of their lives. Delayed loss may start at any time between the age of thirty and the onset of old age; it tends to be confined to the temples.

THE CAUSES OF BALDNESS

We are beginning to have some idea of what causes this phenomenon which is the source of so much anxiety to so many people.

NERVOUS CAUSES

There is one cause which appears to be common to both sexes.

The bald man is frequently tense, anxious and irritable, the sort of man who thinks, reflects, questions his motives; whereas baldness is very rare in primitive people, who don't have problems of conscience or overtax their brains.

Until the beginning of the last war, few women had careers, with all the responsibilities, burdens and worries that go with them, and their hair seldom fell out before old age. But in the past twenty-five years, cases of delayed alopecia in women have increased dramatically. One can't help thinking that there must be a connection between this fact and the profound changes which have taken place in the status and condition of women over the same period. It's almost as though modern women have achieved political, social and professional equality at the price of a luxuriant head of hair.

The possibility of such a connection is particularly fascinating, since it highlights an aspect of the problem of baldness which may have been overlooked.

Not all forms of progress have the happiest consequences for human beings. It brings new burdens, a new way of life, a new rhythm of existence, all of which have strong repercussions on the equilibrium and reactions of that extraordinary network, the central nervous system, upon which the responsibility of supervising and regulating all the functions of the organism devolves. Looked at in this way, baldness could be seen as a kind of 'disease of modern civilisation'.

It will, of course, be objected that not all human beings in our culture, male or female, lose their hair.

HEREDITARY CAUSES

But other factors intervene at this point.

Plainly, heredity counts for a good deal in men: a boy whose father is bald, or both of whose male grandparents are bald, is an obvious candidate for baldness. But to be a candidate isn't to be doomed: should his grandparents on his mother's side have kept their hair, he may equally well inherit this tendency. That is why it is not uncommon to find two brothers, one of whom is bald and the other not.

All the same, when an adolescent begins to lose his hair and has a bald father, the outlook is poor.

Heredity is a less evident factor in women; but even here one often discovers that the mother, aunt or grandmother of a woman with thinning hair suffered from the same problem.

HORMONAL CAUSES

That being said, despite the importance of hereditary factors, the constitutional cause of baldness, as in seborrhea and hirsutism, is the male hormone.

It has been claimed, in this context, that the pill can cause hair-loss in women. This generalisation doesn't hold water; it can only be applied to the type of contraceptive pill which contains a derivative of the male hormone, and even then only when a predisposition exists, as I have emphasised before: just as the male hormone doesn't cause all women to grow body-hair, neither does it cause all women who take it to lose hair from their head.

In a given individual it doesn't even affect all parts of the scalp-hair: in other words, not all the hairs on the head react in the same way to the factors which influence their development.

Experimental hair 'transplants' have shown that the crux of the problem lies in the hair-follicle itself.

As I pointed out earlier, the circlet of hair, the sole remaining ornament of the otherwise completely bald head, never falls out. But when a tuft of hair is taken from the occipital zone at the back of the head, together with the intact 'core' of scalp-tissue in which it was rooted, and this is transplanted to a bald patch, the transplant will 'take' and its hair continue to grow as well in its new location as in its original one.

We can therefore conclude from this that it is not local causes such as the circulation of the scalp, or general causes such as the total amount of hormones circulating in the blood, which have in themselves provoked the loss of hair in the bald areas, but *an abnormal sensitivity of the hair in these areas* to the factors in question. Were this not the case, there is no reason why the transplanted hair should not suffer the same fate as the hair it replaced: the reason it does not is because it reacts differently.

We are beginning to be able to identify the extremely complicated mechanisms which control the activity of the cells of the hair-root as well as the cells of the sebaceous glands.

The reason why the same cause will produce diametrically opposite results on the hair of the scalp and the body, on the other hand, remains a mystery; why, for example, should the male hormone cause masculine type hair to grow on a woman's stomach, breasts and face, and the hair on her head to fall out? The day we understand that, we shall have gone a long way towards finding an effective treatment for baldness.

Even less do we understand why the identical hormonal stimulation should affect the sebaceous glands but not the hair in some people, and the reverse in others, when both hair and sebaceous glands are focal points of those same hormones. Closely-linked anatomically, their functions controlled by the same regulating mechanism, the hair and the sebaceous glands nevertheless react independently, contrary to all logical expectation. They are independent to the extent that I consider the classic conception of seborrheic alopecia to be completely erroneous.

Alopecia may develop without there being any sign of seborrhea, while at the same time plenty of people have oily scalps without losing so much as a single hair. The two phenomena can co-exist without one being obliged to establish a relationship of cause and effect between them.

It might be objected that hair-loss is greater when combined with seborrhea. This is true, but it is the explanation of this phenomenon which is wrong: in my opinion, it is not the seborrhea which causes the hair to fall out. If baldness develops more quickly when seborrhea is present, it is because the disorders responsible are sufficiently acute to accelerate the destruction of the hair-follicle and interfere with the secretion of the sebaceous glands *at one and the same time.*

Merely to treat the seborrhea, therefore, does not increase one's chances of impeding the progress of baldness in a man or alopecia in a woman; and there is a clear distinction between the problem of hair loss and that of the condition of the hair which, like the skin, can either be normal, too oily, dried-up or affected by age.

THE BASES OF TREATMENT FOR HAIR LOSS

Even when it is practicable, the treatment of hair loss is always prolonged, exacting and difficult. It should therefore never be undertaken unless there is a very strong case for it.

There is obviously a clinical case for treatment when the thinning of the hair is clearly noticeable. But it's a different matter when the would-be patient's hair shows little, if any, evidence of thinning, because one can't always take his word for it. Such is the shame many people attach to growing bald that they deliberately exaggerate their symptoms for fear of not being taken seriously.

One also comes across cases where the patient's hair appears to be naturally rather thin, or where the hair loss is temporary and alarming rather than potentially serious. In the first instance he wants to know whether or not his thin hair is in the process of getting thinner; in the second, whether or not his temporary hair loss will become permanent.

In such cases it is impossible to give an answer based on clinical observation alone. As I've already said, what counts is not so much the degree of hair loss as the rate of re-growth. And while it is easy to see how much hair is falling out, it is impossible to see, other than along the hairline, how much is re-growing.

There used to be no way out of this impasse: either one had to wait and see, which certainly didn't appeal to the anxious patient, or else one embarked on an all-purpose treatment without any real justification. Clearly, neither of these approaches was satisfactory.

THE 'TRICHOGRAM'

A few years ago a laboratory test called a trichogram was devised which has solved this dilemma and enables a clear case for treatment to be established: it is based on the fact that there are three stages in the life of a hair: growth – slowing-down – rest, as I explained at the beginning of this chapter.

Seven days after shampooing – this time-lapse is essential to avoid all possibility of error – a tuft of forty or so hairs is taken, by means of a single tug with hair tweezers, from the three key zones of the scalp: the temples, the frontal zone and the crown. Each tuft is spread out, fixed to a glass slide and examined under a microscope. Since the hair-bulb has a characteristic appearance at each stage of development, a count is made of those hairs in the growth phase, those in the resting phase and those in the slowing-down phase. And one then establishes the percentage for each category: we know that, for every hundred hairs, a person with a balanced hair-growth will have no more than fifteen hairs in the resting phase. Thus we can easily distinguish a temporary, occasional hair loss from a potentially serious one, and in the latter case discover precisely how serious it is. The greater the number of resting hairs, the worse the prospects for the future.

This analytical technique is reliable and its results can be verified and reproduced: that is to say that, in a given individual, several trichograms carried out in quick succession will give exactly the same results. Not only does it enable one to make a precise diagnosis in cases where this is not possible by clinical observation alone, but it enables one to forecast future developments.

For example, in a case of an adolescent aged fifteen or sixteen whose hair has not yet started to fall out but whose father is bald, the trichogram will tell him the worst or put his mind at rest. If the verdict is unpleasant, he at least knows where he stands; not only that, but the number of resting hairs enables one to decide whether or not treatment is worthwhile: above a certain percentage, any attempt is doomed to failure.

Personally, I wouldn't dream of undertaking treatment without first doing a trichogram, any more than I would think of continuing with it without periodically checking its results by further trichograms. The impressions one gathers from clinical observation during treatment for alopecia, for instance, are notoriously inaccurate: it's almost impossible to judge its effects with any certainty for several months, or, if one notices any improvement, to know whether this is due to the treatment or to a spontaneous lull in the hair-loss such as often occurs in all types of baldness.

Thanks to the trichogram, one can establish whether a treatment is effective and worth pursuing or modifying, or whether it would be better to abandon the idea of treatment altogether. All this demands the most careful reflection and weighing-up; many patients are so obsessed with their problem that they are plunged into gloom, if not depression. It's all the more important, therefore, that both summing-up and verdict should have a sound basis.

It's not much consolation for a young man to be told that a high, domed forehead gives him an intellectual air, or that baldness is a sign of virility and certainly no obstacle where women are concerned, when all he wants is a career on the stage as a juvenile lead, or if he sees himself as a dynamic, handsome, clear-eyed, bronzed young businessman with the requisite glossy head of hair.

A philosophical acceptance of the inevitable is, alas, nearly

N

always the only solution to the problems of masculine baldness. All one can offer, at present, is experimental therapy of dubious effectiveness in the hope, nearly always unfulfilled, of achieving some improvement.

HAIR TRANSPLANTS

Once they have become bald, those who refuse to resign themselves to the inevitable can have recourse to transplants: cylindrical cores of hair-bearing skin about five millimetres in diameter are taken under a local anaesthetic from the occipital zone. Using the same instrument, something like a 'punch', holes of the same dimension are prepared to receive the transplants in the frontal zone to be refurbished. The art of the operator lies in knowing how and where to place them. Some specialists can transplant a hundred or more tufts in a single session, and, within a few sessions, achieve a satisfactory refurbishment of the bald parts of the scalp.

In the zone from which the tufts were taken, the holes heal over and are hidden by the remaining hair, so that all trace of them rapidly disappears. In the treated zone, however, the marks of the operation remain visible for some time; it's advisable to wear a wig until they have vanished.

Women are luckier than men in that they never go completely bald; furthermore, there are treatments available to women which are denied to men. It must be emphasised once again, however, that these treatments are not always effective.

THE PILL

Basically, treatment consists of prescribing courses of the pill, the same type as that used in the treatment of seborrhea, over prolonged periods of eighteen months to two years.

In addition, as hair-loss in women is never permanent, one can try to stimulate new growth in place of temporarily lost hairs with the use of injections of tissue, embryo or placenta extracts. These have been an unqualified success in some cases.

EXTERNAL TREATMENT

The same extracts, when applied externally, have no effect because they cannot penetrate the epidermal barrier. And no more effective external treatment has yet been discovered.

I repeat: for the present, there is no cream, lotion or other concoction which has the slightest effect on either feminine alopecia or masculine baldness.

I well remember an advertising campaign of some twenty years ago: it proclaimed the merits of a scalp-lotion which made the hair grow. As proof, it showed photographs of a man before and after treatment. In fact, the man in question was suffering from an extreme case of *alopecia areata*, a disorder which looks like baldness but is in fact quite unconnected with it: *alopecia areata* is the result of sudden hair-loss in round patches which may occur anywhere on the scalp; it's caused by a disorder which affects the circulation of the blood in the tiny vessels which nourish the hair matrix and which is nervous in origin; except in a few severe cases, happily rare, the lost hair is always replaced by new growth, often without treatment, and the more you leave it alone, the quicker and better it grows. Needless to say, the miracle lotion failed to produce a single hair and, fortunately, it vanished from circulation along with the illusions it had created.

MASSAGE

It's a long time since I had any faith in the virtues of massage. It may be very pleasant when expertly done, but its effectiveness ends there. Its apologists claim that it improves the circulation and 'loosens' the scalp.

If hair fell out because of lack of circulation due to the scalp adhering too tightly to the skull, it would be a different matter.

Not only do some people believe this, but they claim to obtain results by cutting the fibrous skein which covers the skull like a cap and, being closely interwoven with the scalp, keeps it firmly in place over the bones.

At the same time, other people are firmly convinced that the true cause of alopecia is an excess flow of blood and that the remedy is to ligature the superficial temporal artery.

These diametrically opposed theories seem to me very disturbing, both because they contradict one another and because the far-fetched solutions they propose take no account of the essential causes, nervous and hormonal, of the disorder—causes which are no longer disputed by serious practitioners but which we still don't know how to treat.

While we cannot expect of any external treatment that it will prevent our hair thinning or stop us from going bald, we are nevertheless entitled to expect that it won't complicate matters by causing additional disorders and that, in the long run, it will help to maintain the hair-shaft in the best possible condition.

THE BASES OF HYGIENIC AND COSMETIC CARE OF THE SCALP AND HAIR

The efficacy or harmfulness of products designed for the care of the hair is limited to the surface of the scalp and the hair-shafts emerging from it, while their aim is to maintain or create healthy-looking hair that is shiny without being greasy, supple and resistant to breakage.

In order to judge the condition of hair and scalp — naturally, you can't talk of one without the other — they should never be examined after having been recently shampooed. What I said earlier about the examination of the skin applies equally well here. After it has just been shampooed, seborrheic hair is indistinguishable from normal hair. At least twenty-four to thirty-six hours, in the worst cases, must elapse before the oily coating re-forms and one can see how bad it is.

I never accept a patient's word for it that her hair is as oily as she says it is, and it frequently transpires that when I examine her under proper conditions, that is to say four or five days after shampooing, I find that her seborrhea is mild or moderate, presenting very different problems from that of acute seborrhea.

SEBORRHEA OF THE SCALP

More people come to me with seborrhea of the scalp than with any other condition; women in particular detest having their hair glued together by sebum into heavy oily strands; and the thinner their hair, the worse it looks; thinning hair on its own can be disguised by a hair-piece or a suitable hair-style, but you can't do anything with hair that is both thin and oily: it looks dreadful.

The seborrhea doesn't have to be acute in order to make the hair look unpresentable; a very mild condition is enough. And here one must proceed with caution: mild seborrhea might simply be the result of improper care which, instead of improving matters, only makes them worse.

The story is nearly always the same:

One day Mrs Smith thinks that her hair looks dull and lank; it hasn't been washed for six days. She normally shampoos it once a week, having been told this was about right. But she decides that it will look nicer if she washes it every six days instead. A few weeks later she's surprised to find that five days after it has been shampooed, her hair looks as dull and lank as it used to after six days. She therefore consults the girl behind the cosmetics counter, or her local chemist, explains the trouble and is given a shampoo for oily hair. After the third or fourth time she washes it, her hair is greasier than ever within five days. Desperate ills call for desperate remedies: she takes to washing her hair every five days. Things go from bad to worse. After four days, she can do nothing with it; she returns to the chemist and asks his advice. Needless to say, he recommends a sulphur lotion for oily hair. This is the last straw! By now, she is in the grip of the chain-reaction I call 'reactive seborrhea': the more she de-greases her scalp, the greasier it becomes, and she has ended up with hair that is oilier, twenty-four hours after shampooing, than it was when she used to wash it once a week.

When seborrhea is limited to the scalp, therefore, one must beware of jumping to the conclusion that it is hormonal in origin: 50 per cent of such cases, in my experience, are mainly, if not wholly, the result of using strong detergent preparations too frequently, the worst offenders being those shampoos designed for oily hair and pretentiously labelled 'medicated' shampoos. Personally, I call them 'irritant' shampoos.

In my innocence, I thought that nothing could surpass such rubbish. I was wrong. I have discovered new heights of absurdity in something called 'treatment' lacquer. Never in my wildest dreams did I imagine that hair could be treated with a lacquer. I had always thought of lacquer as an ingenious and useful way of keeping hair in place, a distinct improvement on the old-fashioned brilliantines. Little did I realise what was going on under my very nose!

The moral of this story is that hair, be it oily, normal or dried up, should be washed in products containing as little detergent as possible. The most suitable, from the point of view of their ingredients, are those labelled for 'dry' or 'lifeless' hair. But even these should not be used too frequently. I tell patients that they must try and hold out for six days, using a dry shampoo on the second and fourth days if necessary.

Best of all they could eschew all types of shampoos and clean their hair with mud packs like Tunisian women who don't know the meaning of reactive seborrhea and dried-up hair!

DRIED-UP HAIR

Hair can become dried-up because the sebaceous glands in the scalp are not secreting enough sebum; but more often than not it is the result of dehydration of the hair-shafts due to over-washing —in other words, the harm caused by over-enthusiasm and too much detergent. Like the keratin in the horny layer of the epidermis, the keratin in the hair is absorbent. But whereas the horny layer obtains its water directly from the cellular layers of the epidermis, the hair-shaft, which lies outside the skin apart from the short section within the follicular canal, is entirely dependent on the water which it can get from the exterior—the sweat, the humidity in the atmosphere and the various preparations applied to it.

The sensitivity of hair to variations in humidity is so great that hairs are used in hygrometers, instruments used in the measurement of atmospheric humidity. The damper the hair, the more it will lie flat and go limp; thus in people who perspire on the scalp, however mildly, the hair looks heavy and lank, and is easily mistaken for oily hair. Conversely, if it becomes dried-up, it shrinks, stiffens, and becomes brittle and hard to manage. This condition is a sure sign that, through improper care, the hair has been deprived of its normal film of sebum which is its only protection against dehydration.

Here, at last, we may legitimately talk of moisturising preparations; but, alas, none exists, and all I can do is advise the use of those preparations least likely to dehydrate the keratin in the hair-shaft, such as lipo-protein shampoos.

DANDRUFF

As we have seen, the most that we can expect from hair-cosmetics is that they should be harmless.

Where dandruff is concerned, however, there is an exception. By dandruff, I don't mean the scurf caused by strong detergents which irritate the horny layer of the scalp as they do any other part of the skin, whether seborrheic or not. This will disappear as soon as you stop using the offending product.

True dandruff is bacterial in origin; it can be compared to rough, dry patches on the skin. It will respond to certain shampoos and lotions which owe their genuine anti-dandruff properties to extremely active anti-bacterial ingredients: to these preparations alone, out of the entire range of hygienic and cosmetic products, can the words 'medicated' or 'treatment' be applied.

SPLIT AND BROKEN HAIR

Leaving aside seborrhea and dandruff (which are in fact diseases of the scalp affecting the hair), damage to the hair itself, resulting in its becoming dried up and broken, is less common than might be imagined considering the ways in which it is abused.

When a hair-shaft breaks longitudinally we say that it has 'split'. This condition occurs only in hair of a certain length and then only at the end, in other words, in the oldest part of the hair-shaft. The damage is purely local and doesn't mean that there's anything wrong with the hair itself. The only solution is to cut it off above the split end.

A true break, or horizontal fracture, of the hair-shaft can be the result of a badly-done permanent wave; this is increasingly rare now that hairdressers have become more knowledgeable. But it can also happen as a result of the oxydising agents used in bleaching, a traumatic procedure such as back-combing or combing out lacquered hair, or the absurd process of giving it 'a hundred strokes of the brush' every day.

Notwithstanding all these practices, accidents are rare and the hair stands up well to such abuses. I know women who have been bleaching and back-combing their hair for thirty years without apparent ill-effect.

Sometimes, however, this impressive resistance crumbles, and the hair becomes as brittle as straw. Oddly enough, it never seems to occur to people that it could have anything to do with the way they treat their hair: they blame poor health or being generally run-down.

What people fail to realise is that a hair-shaft, being an inert substance, cannot become damaged throughout its length as the result of internal causes in the space of a few days, or even a few weeks. Internal causes affect the hair-root, the first visible sign of damage being limited to the base of the shaft. When the entire length of the shaft is affected, you may be sure that the cause is external.

The culprit is never hair-dye; this is a common misapprehension. True, the colouring agents in hair-dyes may be harmful, but in a quite different way: they are powerful allergens, so much so that hairdressers should always do a patch-test behind the ear forty-eight hours beforehand.

As I have said, an allergy is an acquired phenomenon. Depending on the circumstances, the substance and the area affected, the reaction can either occur immediately or be delayed. The fact that a product may have been handled for years without ill-effect is no guarantee that you are immune to it: quite the contrary.

Equally, the fact that a woman has had her hair dyed ten, twenty or even a hundred times without incident doesn't mean that on the hundred and first occasion she won't develop an acute eczema within hours.

Eczema resulting from hair-dyes is always accompanied by violent itching, redness and swelling of the scalp, face and ears, and by oozing. The hair itself is unaffected: from that point of view, of all the products used in hairdressing, dyes are the least harmful.

5 Disfiguring conditions of parts of the body

It was while attempting to repair the mutilated faces of the wounded during the First World War that surgeons realised that they could perform a useful service in correcting not only the damage resulting from man's destructive folly but also nature's errors. Many a face might have been attractive had it not been disfigured by a disproportionately large or deformed nose. And it was indeed to the nose that nascent cosmetic surgery first turned its attention.

Whether the fault lay in the skill of the surgeons themselves or in a general reluctance to accept the idea, the fact is that fifty years ago this type of surgery was regarded with supercilious disapproval, if not mistrust.

Although things have improved considerably since then, and although cosmetic surgery has become a small part of the much wider field of plastic surgery, to this day the general public and even the medical world often seem to have only a vague and ill-informed notion of its methods and objectives.

Plastic surgery is concerned with the shapes and contours of the human body. These being largely determined by the cutaneous envelope, it follows that the skin is the plastic surgeon's first objective. We have already seen what it can do by smoothing out wrinkles, tautening the face and the neck and correcting drooping eyelids.

But the role of cosmetic surgery is not limited to tightening the skin in order to 'repair the ravages of time'. By working on those structures — fat, bones, cartilages, muscles — whose proportions and volume dictate the surface contours, it can also correct congenital abnormalities and the deformities which occur incidentally in the course of a lifetime.

Thus plastic surgery at once corrects, repairs and reconstructs, as it seeks to restore balance and harmony to our outer shell.

It is an important branch of skin treatment, as heart surgery is an important branch of heart treatment. And just as cardiologists and heart surgeons work closely together, so dermatologists and plastic surgeons find themselves in constant collaboration, to the great benefit of both disciplines.

Surgery which aims at re-creating a missing part of the anatomy, such as an amputated finger, and surgery which uses skin or bone grafts to repair extensive wounds, whether accidental or surgical, are outside the scope of this book. I shall limit myself to describing the possibilities offered by modern 'corrective surgery', commonly known as 'cosmetic surgery'. Unfortunately, unlike all other kinds of treatment I have mentioned so far, cosmetic surgery is available only to a privileged minority; but let us hope that the day will soon come when it will be within the reach of all.

People still occasionally sneer at it; less and less, it is true; such operations are a waste of time, some say: people should put up with the looks that nature gave them. This is to misunderstand completely the effect a malformation can have on the personality of someone for whom it amounts to a disfigurement. No one has the right to dismiss as negligible the psychological effects and possible repercussions of physical deformity. On the other hand, it would be equally wrong to exaggerate the psychological aspects: many people with physical deformities are perfectly well-adjusted and go through life unaffected by them.

Thus, confronted with an aesthetic problem and the needs of his patient, the plastic surgeon must act as mediator; he alone can be the judge of the possibilities and the limitations of his technique, a question not merely of surgical skill, but of eye and taste, and he must know what to refuse.

The principal areas on which he exercises his skill are the face, breasts and stomach.

THE CORRECTION OF FACIAL DEFORMITIES

Cosmetic surgery of the face includes: lifting, neck surgery, eyelid surgery (all of which I have already described in detail), nose surgery and ear surgery.

While the elderly tend to seek assistance from the first three of these operations, nose-remodelling is much in demand among younger people.

NOSE SURGERY (RHINOPLASTY)

Whether congenital or the result of an accident, nasal imperfections vary considerably: from the bony, fixed part to the mobile, cartilaginous tip; from the general positioning to the length; from the degree of curve to the width of base, bridge or tip; from the relationship to the upper lip to the angle with the forehead. In theory, a well-proportioned face is one in which the distance from the base of the nose to the chin is equal to that between the base of the nose and the base of the forehead.

In a child, the tip of the nose is round and uptilted. The nose straightens as you grow up, and lengthens with age, the point tending to grow down towards the upper lip. Shortening a nose thus makes a face look younger, while raising and rounding the tip gives it a childish expression.

When it is properly planned and carried out, rhinoplasty is a straightforward operation. But it also makes great demands on the surgeon's artistic skill.

There was a time when you could tell the surgeon from the type of nose he had given his client. A patient went through life parading 'so-and-so's' nose, not necessarily the one that suited him best. The new generation of surgeons, I'm glad to say, are prepared to take more trouble and have abandoned the 'off-the-peg' nose for the made-to-measure variety demanding greater talent and mastery of technique.

In theory, there is no nasal deformity which cannot be corrected. In practice, the operation should not be done when it is obvious that, however technically and aesthetically perfect the result, there would be no real benefit because of the unpromising nature of the surrounding features: in some cases a pretty nose would only accentuate the faults in the rest of the face. One would also try to persuade someone against having the operation where the imperfection is more imaginary than real, or when the desired shape seems obviously unsuitable.

On the other hand, there are occasions when one might advise more extensive remodelling than the patient had in mind: to shorten a long, hooked nose in a face with a prominent or receding chin, for instance, would be little improvement, aesthetically speaking, to the balance of the face as a whole. It then becomes necessary to combine it with a chin operation; and a chin can easily be taken back, by resecting, or 'paring down', the lower jaw, or brought forward, by doing a bone-graft. These operations are only performed on adults who have stopped growing, in order to avoid the necessity for further corrections later in life.

EAR SURGERY

However, there is one operation which can and even should be done in childhood: the stitching-back of so-called bat ears. Children can be pitilessly cruel and a visible deformity is an invitation to teasing and jibes. The child should be rescued at the earliest possible moment from persecution which may affect him for life. Between seven and eight is the best age for stitching back the ears. It is a straightforward, routine operation, which causes little discomfort and can be done under a local anaesthetic; it has excellent, permanent results.

DEFORMITIES OF THE BREASTS

Symbol of femininity, the breast is an organ of complex structure and hence vulnerability: first and foremost, it's a gland whose function is to secrete milk after childbirth, and whose collecting ducts flow into the nipple; the latter is a sensitive, erectile structure, capable of swelling or hardening when stimulated, as by suckling. It is also an erogenous zone which plays a considerable part in love-making.

The mammary gland, which may be large or small, is enclosed by a mass of fatty tissue, more abundant in some people than others.

Glands and fat are enclosed within an envelope of skin, and the firmness of the breast depends on the relationship between this envelope and its content. If the envelope is nicely full, the breast is firm and taut; if it is overstretched, or if the fatty mass dissolves, the breast becomes slack and soft.

It also depends on a belt of fibrous tissue called the breast suspensory ligament which is joined at one end to the connective fibres attached to the clavicle and at the other to the fibrous envelope of the great pectoral muscle. When the suspensory ligament is taut and securely attached to the muscles, the breast is held firmly in place against the thoracic cage. If there is a slackening of the ligaments, or of the great pectoral muscle, the breast will obey the laws of gravity and drop to the base of the thorax.

The perfect breast is seen only in the normal adolescent. Women who retain firm, well-set breasts after adolescence are the exception; variations in weight, menstrual problems, pregnancies, lack of muscular tone, soon take their toll; place a pencil in the fold beneath the breast of a woman over thirty and it will have an annoying tendency to stay there.

Everything that I have said so far applies to the development of breasts which were normal to begin with. In some cases, however, the breasts grow so large after puberty that they amount to a positive infirmity — not merely from the point of view of looks but because their weight tends to drag the body forwards, imposing a permanent and abnormal strain on the muscles of the back and loins which a bra can do little to relieve. In other cases, the breasts never develop at all and differ little from the barely perceptible mounds on a man's chest.

Whether it's a question of huge pendulous breasts, empty sagging flat breasts or diminutive breasts, they can all be treated by corrective surgery.

Surgery is the sole means whereby deformed or malformed breasts can be restored to their proper shape, size and position. No chemical products, whether in the form of ampoules, creams or lotions, no mechanical or electrical paraphernalia allied to the use of massage, vibrations or water-spray, the claims for which are as preposterous as they are mendacious, have the least effect.

Such advertisements are a great temptation to women with breast deformities: 'Improvement guaranteed in two months', 'firmer figure in three weeks' they proclaim, and even go so far as to guarantee a refund 'if not delighted', knowing perfectly well that they run no risk of their bluff being called. What woman is going to complain that she has been hoaxed? It would be tantamount to admitting publicly to badly-shaped breasts and to having allowed herself to be gulled!

Even medical preparations based on hormones, rubbed into the breasts in order to try to stimulate the enlargement of the mammary gland, gives inconsistent, mediocre, and purely temporary results.

Breast surgery is a great deal more complicated than facial surgery. Not that it is difficult for a skilled surgeon to make a pair of matching, symmetrical breasts; but the post-operative period involves considerable discomfort for days or even weeks, the sensitivity of the nipple may be either diminished or lost, temporarily or permanently, and, lastly, there is a tendency to abnormal scar formation.

DROOPING OR OVERDEVELOPED BREASTS

Breasts may be lifted in a number of different ways. Whatever the technique employed, it necessitates an incision all round the nipple, since this must be moved.

Depending on the volume and shape of the breast, the size of the mammary gland and the constitution of the skin, one may be able to manage with a single incision which will leave an oblique scar on the outer side of the breast; more often than not, one is obliged to make incisions which leave an anchor-shaped scar whose stem (or shank, in nautical terms) descends vertically from the nipple to the fold beneath the breast and whose cross-bar extends from the edge of the sternum (the bone in the centre of the chest to which the ribs are attached) on one side to the armpits on the other.

Although one could hardly call the resulting scars negligible, they are largely compensated for by the unquestionable advantages of the operation.

Nevertheless, anyone contemplating the operation should be warned that she will keep these visible scars for the rest of her life: they will be red for some months, then pale gradually until, once white, they cease to be disfiguring – provided, that is, that they don't become thick or distended.

ABNORMAL SCARS

These two contingencies are fairly common: if the surgeon has found it necessary to exercise a strong pull on the flaps of skin in order to position the breast correctly, the scar, always a weak point, will have a tendency to enlarge.

Moreover, the chest is one of the zones of the body most prone to the formation of the hard red thick scars known as 'hypertrophic' scars. A hypertrophic scar does not develop immediately; all seems well for six to eight weeks after the operation, then, suddenly, the line of the scar alters: it swells and becomes cord-like in appearance. At this point, two things may happen:

1 Either this development is short-lived, the dimension of the slightly raised cord reaching no more than two to three millimetres in diameter, when the scar will 'pull' slightly, which may be uncomfortable but not painful; or

2 It will continue to evolve, causing the scar to increase in volume, more in some places than others, when it will itch, become sensitive and even painful; this is what is called a 'keloid'.

A keloid is much more of a nuisance than a simple hypertrophic scar: while the latter should clear up of its own accord within eighteen months or two years, a keloid is self-perpetuating and never clears up spontaneously.

The main problem with abnormal scars is their total unpredictability. Some scars will become hypertrophic or keloid for only part of their length, abnormal stretches alternating with normal ones. Some people never develop them, others, only after their second operation; so that if you do an operation to improve a simple enlarged scar, there is a risk of replacing it with a hypertrophic one.

The treatment of abnormal scars is difficult but not impossible. The earlier it is undertaken the better the chances of success. But on no account should a keloid be removed by surgery; the result can be disastrous: nine times out of ten a new keloid will form, far bigger than the first.

The chest does not have a monopoly of abnormal scars. The stomach, too, is very prone to them. On the face they are much rarer and occur, if at all, as simply hypertrophic scars in front of the ears, the zone which suffers the greatest traction during lifting. As a rule, the scars behind the ears merely become distended.

But where scars are concerned, there is never any absolute rule. I have twice seen enormous keloids in young boys who had had their ears stitched back – an operation involving the remodelling of cartilage with the minimum of traction.

In fact, there is only one area where you never find abnormal cicatrisation, and that is on the eyelids.

With these reservations, breast-surgery can transform the lives of some women, especially as its results are lasting – an important factor when you consider that it is not an operation one would willingly undergo more than once.

UNDERDEVELOPED BREASTS

Underdeveloped breasts present a quite different problem: there is no physical strain involved, as in overdeveloped breasts. As far as social life goes, their lack of size can be camouflaged by artificial padding. It is the degree to which they make a woman feel psychologically or sexually inferior that leads her to seek an operation.

This consists of an implant of suitable size and shape inserted on the underside of the breast and composed of substances acceptable to the organism, that is, substances which won't be rejected by its protective mechanism.

In the past, attempts were made to inject substances behind the mammary gland. In theory, this was deceptively easy: all you had to do was to open the breasts. But there were some unpleasant surprises in store: the substances, pulled down by gravity, spread into the subcutaneous tissue and ended up in the lower abdomen, not the ideal location for breasts!

Daring experiments in corrective surgery and dermatology to boost nature's own efforts are all very well at times, but they should never be done blindly.

DISFIGUREMENTS OF THE ABDOMEN

Surgery to correct the effects of wear and tear on the abdominal wall is not confined to the problems of age, any more than that of the breasts. Like the breasts, the abdomen may be damaged prematurely by repeated pregnancies, or by slimming diets for corpulence; it can also 'collapse' following an operation (this is called eventration).

For the patient in search of a solution to any of these problems, there is no alternative to surgery at present. No cream can retighten distended tissues.

What she hopes for is a flat stomach free from visible scars on the midriff. What she will get is a smooth stomach, but not necessarily a flat one; the surface relief of the abdomen depends not only on the amount of subcutaneous fat, but also on the amount of fat surrounding the peritoneum, the membrane lining the abdominal cavity.

As for scars, these necessarily vary with the type of deformity and the kind of operation this dictates.

In most cases the operation must be preceded by a slimming diet in order to bring down the weight to somewhere near the ideal. This ensures the best possible recovery as well as the best cicatrisation, and it goes without saying that the diet must be continued after the operation in order to avoid a relapse.

Cosmetic surgery of the abdomen presents fewer difficulties than that of the breasts, and the two operations may usefully be combined. It is highly inadvisable, however, to combine it with surgery of the buttocks or thighs; this is a pity, for the inner face of the upper thigh is a weak point in the musculature and the elasticity of the skin. Full of pitfalls, from visible, delayed and defective scars to extravasations of blood and lymph, cosmetic surgery to the thighs should only be undertaken in exceptional cases, a fact which is not without its attendant problems.

I remember a friend on the beach at Cannes a few years ago. With her re-shaped, firm breasts, successfully-lifted face and neck, youthful, artistically made-up eyelids, restored abdomen and her own natural, unforced vitality, she was very attractive indeed ... as long as one looked no lower than her buttocks: the insides of her sadly withered thighs drooped like flags on a windless day, all the more noticeable for their striking contrast to the rest of her body.

I can understand her surgeon advising her against having this supplementary operation, but I shall never understand why such an intelligent woman should have failed to realise how much better she would have looked in trousers ...

DISORDERS OF THE LEGS

The legs are prone to a number of disorders. As we have seen, they are not only uniquely vulnerable to 'cellulite', but their elastic tissue is weak compared to the rest of the body.

In addition, they are subject to swelling and superficial circullatory disorders.

Any swelling of the legs should be medically investigated, because it may be the result of malfunction of the kidneys, cardiac trouble or deep circulatory disorders.

Superficial circulatory disorders, varicose veins and varicosities, are congenital in origin. Jobs that necessitate standing for long

o

periods, such as hairdressing and dentistry, often trigger them off in people with this predisposition.

Varicose veins are not an exclusively feminine complaint; although they are more common in women, men are by no means exempt.

They rarely occur singly, usually resulting from the dilation of the tiny capillaries of the dermis as in broken veins of the face. These networks of fine red lines which criss-cross the thighs and, in the worst cases, the whole of the legs, are especially unpleasant because of their tendency to spread until they coalesce.

Although varicose veins without finer varicosities are rare, the reverse is not the case: varicosities can exist without visible varicose veins. They can be aggravated by disorders of the ovaries and over-exposure to the sun.

THE TREATMENT OF VARICOSITIES OR BROKEN VEINS IN THE LEGS

Their treatment is less unpleasant and made easier and more effective if it is undertaken as soon as the first signs appear: it is simpler to deal with three or four capillaries than an entire mass. And since we can be sure that those three or four are merely the beginning, it is better not to wait for the inevitable.

They are treated by means of electrolysis, as in broken veins of the face.

This should be done in winter for preference, since while the traces left by electrolysis on the face disappear completely within eight to ten days, the same treatment on the legs, using the identical current and needles and performed by the identical operator, will leave minute scabs which turn into red dots and take two to three months to clear up completely.

It is therefore highly inadvisable to undergo this treatment in May: more than likely you will not be able to bare your legs in August, or, should you do so, pigment may develop at each point of coagulation.

Once cicatrisation is complete, a minute white trace is all that remains of the vanished capillaries.

Despite what people sometimes say, electrolysis is completely effective; but like all treatments of the kind, it requires patience and conscientiousness on the part of the operator and patience and endurance on the part of the patient; in fact, according to people who have experienced both, electrolysis on the legs is more unpleasant than on the face; one more reason for not waiting until things get really bad before embarking upon treatment.

THE TREATMENT OF VARICOSE VEINS

Obviously, when there are varicose veins present, they must be dealt with at the same time; and, if they are bad, they should be treated before the capillaries.

I am more and more in favour of surgery. It is a routine operation with every chance of success; it is also one which never need be repeated: once a vein is removed it will never grow again; whereas the method of injection of sclerosants, which blocks the veins little by little, can be interminable when there are large trunk vessels involved. In principle, therefore, I recommend removing the main vessels by surgery and reserving sclerosant injections for the finishing touches, that is, for the destruction of the remaining small veins.

Properly carried out, these treatments are not merely a great improvement to the appearance of legs disfigured by purple veins, they also bring physical relief by reducing or even entirely removing that heaviness which always accompanies circulatory disorders.

The various medicaments designed to tone up the veins and strengthen the capillary vessels are never enough in themselves; they merely complement dermatological or surgical treatment. They are certainly useful supportive therapy but never really effective unless used regularly over very long periods.

Conclusion

The average standard of looks among white people is not very high: when you look around you on the beach, or in any public place, the spectacle which greets your eyes is hardly edifying.

Age for age, there is a far higher proportion of men with good physique in some African ethnic groups, and feminine beauty among the Eurasians of Indonesia.

For the majority of Westerners, the possession of an attractive physical appearance is an achievement, and a difficult one. It entails (a) a knowledge of the means required to attain this objective, hence a search for information; (b) an effort in order to succeed, hence will-power; (c) constant vigilance to maintain it, hence perseverance.

This raises an immediate question: does one's external appearance warrant the expenditure of so much time, trouble and energy? It seems to me that the answer is yes: beauty is surely an asset to oneself and a pleasure to others.

Such is its magnetic power that every generation throws up thousands of copies of the individuals who embody its idea. This may not testify to human originality, but the sight of a swarm of little Bardots, as long as the imitations were reasonably faithful, was by no means disagreeable.

However, beauty is not everything, and to make it an end in itself is to lose all sense of proportion. There are some types of beauty so unhealthy and perverse as to make one yearn for ugliness, and some types of warm-hearted ugliness far preferable to the coldness of some beauties.

Beauty is a snare and a delusion unless accompanied by physical and mental balance, that complete state of well-being which is called health and which, in my view, is more important than anything else.

Indeed, it's the radiance emanating from a healthy child or adolescent that makes them seem beautiful even when they are not, and because of this that youth constitutes a frame of reference and a value which is the envy of those who are no longer young. But there can be no beauty at whatever age without health, and the beauty of youth turns into a sinister myth when one is confronted with a twenty-year-old drug addict.*

If one accepts that health is the passport to true beauty, one cannot avoid the conclusion that, despite all the progress achieved in both the medical and the social spheres, industrial societies, which generate so much pollution and nervous tension, do not make its acquisition easy.

It is true that, in a country such as ours, people appear to live better today than did their forebears, in that they have greater comfort and security. They need no longer fear the sort of epidemics which once decimated whole populations — and did so until relatively recently when one considers that the last outbreak of plague occurred in India in 1894, spread to China, reached the Pacific Coast of America, then North Africa, and made itself felt as far as Portugal before subsiding in 1912. Nor are they threatened with famine, which is still rife over a considerable area of the globe.

On the other hand, modern Western man is subjected to all the harmful effects of increasing noise, haste and speed, and has become so conditioned to the accelerating rhythm of life that he has carried it over into his leisure activities as well as his work. With no time left for thought or reflection, mesmerised by advertising slogans, dominated by inventions that enslave as much as serve him, he has more and more difficulty in finding or keeping his equilibrium.

In view of all this, one may well ask oneself whether there is not a certain vanity in talking about beauty when what we need above all is to learn, or relearn, how to live. Yet history shows that the desire to beautify the human body dates from remotest antiquity and is to be found in all societies, however precarious their conditions of existence. We have evidence that the Hebrews, who were initiated into the arts of perfumery during their exile in Egypt, subsequently brought their skill and knowledge in this field up to a level hitherto unattained. In the Egypt of the Pharaohs, the art of make-up and the dyeing and waving of hair were already being practised. During their military campaigns around the Mediterranean the Romans discovered these practices and brought them to Rome where they were widely used: all the cosmetics used in the

* See the Appendix for a summary of the skin disorders which may result from drug-taking. (A-B)

daily *toilette* of high-born Roman ladies were specially prepared and applied according to a strict ceremonial by young *cosmetae*, the forerunners of our modern beauticians, and supervised by a specialist who bore the title of *ornatrix*.

In the third century B.C. the Latin poet Ovid wrote in his *Ars Amatoria* or *The Art of Love*:

> Beauty is a gift of the Gods, but how few women can boast of their beauty! It is a gift denied to most. Care will confer charms; but neglected charms will perish, even though they be comparable to those of the Idalain Goddess ...
>
> You know how to borrow the whiteness of ceruse, and lacking blood to blush with, blush by the aid of art. You don't hesitate to use your skill to refurbish brows and cheeks touched by age; nor do you shrink from heightening the gleam of your eyes with filmy ash or saffron from the banks of the limpid Cydnus ...
>
> You will find aids to beauty in a treatise of mine, small in bulk but great in the care I have bestowed on it. You can also find cures for blemishes therein; all my skills are at your disposal.

Two centuries later, Cornelius Celsus, physician to the Emperor Augustus, devoted long passages in his treatise on medicine to plastic surgery, the skin and the hair. Far from declining, interest in cosmetic problems increased, *vide* the numerous works in which they are accorded careful study. In the *Natural History* by the Roman writer and naturalist Pliny the Elder, dating from the first century B.C., there are chapters dealing with the chemistry and botany of perfumes; similarly, in the work of the Greek physician Diocorides, who remained the leading authority until the seventh century, the use of all then known substances, both animal and vegetable, employed in medicine, pharmacology and cosmetology, are described in detail, mud-baths being particularly recommended.

But it was Crito, physician to the Emperor Trojan, who produced the first systematic and scientific study of cosmetics. It appeared in four volumes. The first dealt with the hair and the skin, the second with baths and perfumes, the third with freckles and heat-rash, and the fourth with the various diseases which destroy facial beauty.

Finally, it is to Galen, the greatest physician of the ancient world after Hippocrates, whose work dominated medical thinking until the reign of Louis XIV, that we owe the discovery in the second century of '*cerat*', water mixed with melted beeswax and olive-oil, the ancestor of continuous oily-phase emulsions and the prototype of cold-creams.

Thus, as they have come down to us in these various documents, ancient cosmetological skills were much more extensive than many modern experts, who are tempted to believe they started it all, seem prepared to concede. These encompassed: cosmetics such as cleansing creams, powders, rouges, mascara, eye-shadow and beauty patches as well as remedies for dryness of the teguments, wrinkles, freckles, blackheads, sunburn, warts, scars, double-chins, superfluous hair (depilatories and abrasives) and body odours; and hairdressing accessories such as oils, unguents, bleaches, temporary or permanent hair-dyes, scalp-lotions and medicaments for dandruff, hair-loss and baldness.

As a matter of course this assortment of recipes was used in conjunction with the rules of dietetics and general hygiene laid down by Hippocrates, to which they were merely the complement.

Of course, the results were not always happy: the snake-oil, viper's venom, bear-grease, virgin's urine and ass's milk recommended to combat hair-loss were not wholly successful; and the dyes made from elderberries, or leeches macerated for two months in a lead vase containing red wine and vinegar, dried up and even destroyed the hair.

But at least they show that from the earliest times beauty and health were considered to be interrelated, and that the search for physical perfection has always corresponded to a natural, universal and spontaneous need: the need to please and attract.

And because the knowledge that we are pleasing to other people —something we know from their attitude and expression—is a factor in our own well-being, it is a need which deserves more than ever to be encouraged and satisfied.

How far have we gone towards satisfying it?

The cosmetic industry has made enormous strides in the field of perfumes; the hair-dyes it manufactures are no longer in any way harmful; and the technology of make-up has reached a high level of perfection. On the other hand, the aids proposed to combat hair-loss are no more efficacious today than the snake-oils of two thousand years ago; and if the enormous range of creams and milks are a considerable advancement on Galen's *cerat* and the unguents of the past, they are nevertheless, in terms of what is claimed for them, equally empirical and haphazard.

The pharmaceutical industry, which includes a number of firms that have set up cosmetological departments, has failed to make any impact on this situation, and its products differ from those of the cosmetic industry only in presentation.

As for medicine, apart from plastic surgery whose benefits are still inaccessible to the vast majority, and with the exception of a few tentative, isolated experiments on the part of departmental heads in certain teaching hospitals who have started clinics for cosmetic care – in Lyons, Munich and Prague, for example – the profession is only now beginning to acknowledge the existence of cosmetic dermatology, as I pointed out in my introduction to this book.

One can only regret that this awareness has been so long in coming, since these problems are so manifestly an integral part of the field of public health. The medical profession alone has the knowledge and technical means at its disposal to ensure that cosmetic care and treatment is no longer a luxury but a scientific discipline whereby the quest for beauty can be carried out with safety, moderation and common sense.

The same moderation and common sense which tell us that, despite its importance and the attention it deserves, beauty is only one of many attributes; that charm, grace and attractiveness have their importance too; and that these qualities are much more lasting.

Appendix

TABLE VI   *Skin disorders attributable to the use of drugs*

Any drug	Marijuana	Opium and its derivatives	Cocaine	Barbiturates[3]
Pigmented scars (80% of cases)	Rashes	Itching	Abscesses	Urticaria
	Swelling of the eyelids	Urticaria	Itching	Blisters
Hypertrophic scars (10% of cases)	Acne	Infections	Perforation of the nasal septum	Mottling
	Seborrhea	Oedema[1]		Porphyria[4]
Atrophic scars (3% of cases)	Seborrheic eczema	Eschars[2]	Contact eczema	Purpura[5]
	Folliculitus (rosacea type)			

1   Oedema is a diffuse swelling of the skin.
2   Eschars are necrotic areas of the skin frequently found in the aged who are helpless and bedridden.
3   Barbiturates are normally used as sleeping drugs.
4   Porphyria is a disease due to the presence in the blood of abnormal substances which induce a hyper-sensitivity to light causing the formation of blisters and sores, and a fragilisation of the skin.
5   Purpura is an effusion of blood in the skin, causing small haemorrhagic spots.

Index